# How I escaped dialysis ...

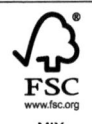

I dedicate this book to my wife Beate, who supported me in every situation unselfishly and without limitation.

Dieter Reinecker

# How I escaped dialysis ...

## The autobiography of a self-healing

**Translated by Christoph Wolters**

Bibliografische Information der Deutschen Nationalbibliothek:
Die Deutsche Nationalbibliothek verzeichnet diese Publikation in der Deutschen Nationalbibliografie;
detaillierte bibliografische Daten sind im Internet über http://dnb.dnb.de abrufbar.

Herstellung und Verlag:
BoD – Books on Demand, Norderstedt

ISBN: 978-3-73921982-0

# I escaped dialysis …

by
Dieter Reinecker

## Introduction

My 'story' is true and has happened as I have written it down here.

In order to substantiate its validity, I have disclosed the lab values regarding creatinine in the appendix. Besides, these were two different laboratories, on the one hand commissioned by the family doctor and on the other hand by two different dialysis centres. These, but also the names of the doctors are known to the publishing company. The names of the doctors in my story are fictitious.

From my health history one cannot, of course, deduce other illness courses. I have made this way alone and in my own responsibility.

It may have been a radical and risky way in many people's views. But it was my way and I am glad to have made it as I did.

I deliberately do not want to give any medical advice or suggest therapies and certainly not advise against medical consultations.

My aim was only to indicate which way I went, and that it is worthwhile to think about it.

### Chapter 1

Do you have a comfortable armchair? If not, a sofa will also do, if all else fails, a bed; a chair is least suitable. The seat should be comfortable. And then you need rest, a lot of rest. I am sitting in the kitchen, on a chair because I am not reading, but writing. In front of me there is an old, but usable laptop. The radio is quiet. My wife is in the sitting room, she wanted to iron a few things, and the television is running aside, but so quietly that I hear nothing. Our children moved out long ago. Strictly speaking, these are her children. I married my wife with two small children. The older one was in the second, the younger in the first school year. I had taken them to my heart from the outset.

I have rest. I also do not belong to the generation which lingers through the streets with earbuds and always runs the risk of being run over. I am nearly fifty-eight years old and it is my first book, at least it should become one. And if you read this, it has indeed become one.

But why do I recommend you to make your-selves at home and to provide for rest? It was rest that helped me to become healthier again.

It has been less than five months. It was the 7th of September, 2010, when I also was sitting at home and sitting and sitting and sitting.

'I want to tell her directly, as she is used to from me, frankly, straight up. How do I start? She knows me too well.'

She asks just by her looks.

Three days before I had gone to the family doctor, and also on this day I went to see him to fetch the lab values.

My wife had asked me to conclude a life insurance policy. We are not so well off, and if anything should happen to me sometime, she wanted to be secured, understandably.

But at my age one has to go to the doctor. I was always healthy, though, and actually had no discomfort. Or did I? Yes, in autumn of last year, in Majorca. I had completely blocked this out; my stomach had ached, even quite violently. There was a dragging pain in the stomach and over the chest, sometimes even in the back. I stopped while taking a walk and bent over forward. This lasted a few seconds. Then it went off again.

And when we went for a walk in Palma, in the harbour, past many boats of 'welfare recipients', we stopped at a harbour café, and I ordered first of all a Canya, a beer, and then another one, until the pain subsided. Stress. Occupational stress well into the holidays. This was my diagnosis then. Alcohol is good. And for the evening, since I really like cooking, I still had to buy some wine. In the morning I already thought of it, so that I would not forget in the course of the day. Yes, so it was, and by the end of those fourteen days I did not have that pain anymore. So it had to have been the stress. Fourteen days are also too short.

So I was sitting there, in the sitting room, no television was on, the radio quiet, and I was thinking. Actually, I still had to write some letters to customers, calculations of construction costs, answer emails. The answering machine – had I switched it on at all? I did not know anymore. My mobile phone was also still off. At the doctor's I had turned it off.

I was accessible to no-one. I had rest. It was quiet around me, very quiet, almost unbearably quiet. Only yesterday I would have cracked a bottle of wine, would have found something in the fridge with my usual security and would have conjured up some delicacies.

For I am very creative in the kitchen. My potato salad is even said to be addictive. I had exactly paid attention to how my granny had prepared it. This granny was the mother of my father, from Upper Silesia. She had even whipped the mayonnaise herself, with yolk and olive oil. But now I am sitting in silence and thinking. Funnily enough, I even feel like eating, but I cannot move, have no motivation to go to the kitchen. I will just tell her that everything is not so bad, and things are never as bad as they seem.

I felt my tears. I began to cry. Immediately I wiped my tears from my face with the sleeve. I did not want to lower my guard towards my wife. But she will notice anyway. Did she know, actually, what creatinine values are? I did not know it quite exactly myself, at that time. But I already had dealt with them.

It was approximately one and a half years ago. I was still with my old family doctor then. I am still to fetch my old medical records from him as well. The new family doctor wanted to look whether there had not been any problem with my values earlier on already. The cause was still absolutely unclear. And I, I had no idea about anything, not the faintest notion. This is additionally frightening.

One and a half years ago, that is meanwhile two years ago, my former family doctor had sent me to a specialist, to a good acquaintance of his, a nephrologist. I heard about this field for the first time then. This is a doctor for the kidneys. I still know exactly how I was sitting in front of my old family doctor, in front of the big black desk; he was behind it, completely in white, even his hair was white, and his easy chair seemed very comfortable and stopped luffing when he looked directly into my eyes and said in a quiet voice:

'You are actually in good health appropriate to your age, only one value worries me...'

Silence.

'The best thing is if I just send you to a specialist. I have some good acquaintance...'

I did not hear the rest anymore at all. The doctor's receptionist, too, suddenly looked round-eyed and was quite serious, somehow mysterious. She pressed a note in my hand, no prescription, just a name with an address. The long hallway of the doctor's office endlessly stretched. I left the doctor's office in a daze. My self-assuredness was gone. Knees, legs, somehow all rubber. I walked through the hall, down the stairs, some people came towards me, I did not perceive them at all. Automatically like a robot, I drove my car, I did not notice that the traffic light went from red to green and I drove off. At that time I had to go directly from the doctor's to the office. I listened to my answering machine. My professional problems had come back to me, and the note with the name of the specialist was well hidden in my purse. I called him from the office. With his assistant I arranged an appointment.

Then, a few days later, I went there. A good half an hour from home in a small place in the country. A plain office, a few elderly ladies in the waiting room. Naturally I immediately went through to the reception and was also, after the collection of my data, sent on when I told her that I am a private patient. A doctor or assistant pressed a big plastic bottle in my hand.

'From 6 or 7 o'clock tonight until the next morning please collect your urine. The first stream, however, is to go into the toilet.'

The fact that you feel funny in this is understandable, so direct and somehow unpleasant. But the instruction was clear and unmistakable. I was just not used to it, and it was a little embarrassing for me, am I also blocked in this regard? In any case, I did not want to show any emotion, took the bottle and said goodbye until tomorrow. I stowed away the big two litre bottle in my briefcase and went home. Once arrived in the flat, I went directly to the bathroom with the briefcase and stowed away, one can probably rather say, I hid the bottle in the little white cupboard under the washbasin.

One day later. Compliant with the demands, I went back to the medical office in the country with the almost full bottle. While driving, I did not listen to any music. I did not want to expose myself to this blaring and stupid drivel, and over and over again these commercials. I am not taken in by these stupid commercials on the radio anyway. Moreover, I turn the radio down if the commercial is announced, or I change the radio station. At my age you prefer listening to WDR or NDR 2; I am sick and tired of the private stations: superficial, commonplaces, childish and kitsch beyond all measure. This has never been my thing. Protected by an opaque Aldi bag avoiding any content, the bottle came into the hands of the assistant. In one week the lab values would be there. After one week I called and also got an appointment with the doctor himself. And then I stood in front of him. He, a true Westphalian, at the sight of whom the Romans would already have fled from the Teutoburg wood, and I, with my 176 cm looking up to him, certainly made a funny impression, and he then laid his big hands on my shoulders and gasped:

'You do look quite healthy. Is anything hurting you?'

I only shook my head timidly and could think of nothing at all. What else he said then, I have forgotten. Two weeks later I received a bill for the amount of 186 euros. I had instantly got the lab values, and they offered nothing new to me either. Somehow then they went yellow in the desk. I never found the note again either. Suppression had completely struck. I have not consulted my former family doctor anymore. What was this nephritic value called again? I had already forgotten the word. And here now I am sitting. Should I blame myself? Whose fault is it then that I thought of everything for nearly two years, just not my lab values? The door lock snapped, steps on the hallway.

'I am here', I shouted.

## Chapter 2

When she entered the sitting room, I got up and looked into her green-blue eyes. In these eyes I saw, at the same time, the eyes of the doctor, his face in outlines and his sombre expression as a whole, and everything at the same time. I turned away irritated and steered towards the hallway in the direction of the bathroom.

'I'll be right back', I shouted and locked behind myself. My face had red spots, and my eyes were dim and moist. I put on my reading glasses and thought I would recognise something yellow. With cold water I moistened my face, dried it up and walked slowly through the narrow, dark hallway full of cupboards to the kitchen. There she was sitting on her usual place at the big wooden table.

'My kidneys are out of order.'

'Very badly?'

'Yes.'

'Do the kidneys not detoxify properly anymore?'

'Somehow. But the values are so bad that Dr von Rothenburg transferred me to the dialysis centre.'

'You will, however, definitely go there. Promised?'

'Of course.'

'Such things must not be taken lightly.'

'I know. So I will go there.'

'Did the doctor say anything about what is the cause?'

'This is inexplicable to him as well. He has really examined everything. Only the lab values showed that the kidneys are not in order, and my blood pressure is probably too high as well, cholesterol is also dramatic.'

My voice became weak and shaky. I lowered my head, felt devastated. She got up, laid one hand on my head and said:

'We'll make it all right. Just go there for the time being, and then we'll see what's going to happen.'

'He also gave me pills, for the high blood pressure, among other things, and something for the cholesterol. I also told him about my professional stress.'

My voice failed. All problems with the customers, authorities and open invoices, the last decades squeezed my head together like in a vice. I would have liked very much to burst out crying. Stress, stress and over and over again stress.

In the evening, after the news broadcast, while we were sitting side by side, her on the daybed, me in the wicker chair, legs stretched out to another wicker chair a little aside of myself, the sound became quieter. Before the sound was completely gone, I heard her voice:

'Good you're not drinking anything now, you have always been drinking too much, and lately it had become more and more. I warned you often enough. You know, this will take revenge sometime. You do know the cases of illness in the circle of acquaintances of our parents. Many are...'

Not only had I heard all that only too well, I knew, meanwhile, every single one with their illness, whether and how he or she was still alive, who had which tumour, only half a bowel left etc. However, if you were never ill yourself, then the others just exaggerated things. I did not see myself as an alcoholic. Last spring I drank no beer or wine for four weeks. I was convinced that no alcoholic is capable of this, and if I have one thing, it is self-restraint.

I still know exactly how I stopped smoking. I had fallen in love with Beate. A 'single' mother with two children, six and seven years old. After a few weeks these were my children, and their mother was the woman of my dreams. At that time I was still smoking. But if I get into this family, I must be a model. As a studied pedagogue, I know that education is useless, because the children will copy everything anyway.

After a temporary contract as a teacher, my employment was not continued, so after a few other unsuccessful attempts at a profession, I went to a building society. At that time I was 41 and meanwhile was a building society representative. An older colleague, to whom I maintained a very amicable contact, was a raw food eater. The first one which I had got to know. Everybody liked him, even though he always stank of garlic. At that time he had recommended me to start with therapeutical fasting and then to begin a new diet with grains, roots and raw vegetables. Moreover, I would then automatically stop smoking. I admired the point about raw food, but it was out of the question for me, did not,. literally, bear any fruit for me. However, I had still kept the thing about therapeutical fasting and not smoking anymore in mind. I still know it exactly.

I smoked my last cigarette on Friday evening, drank a bottle of beer and went for a walk with Dicki, my wire-haired dachshund at that time, but this evening without any detour to the Lenzig or Wolters inn, where I was known and estimated as an interlocutor. No, I had firmly decided to fast now for 36 hours and to drink only mineral water – without carbonic acid, to be sure.

Almost sober, I lay in bed, on my back. Headache. No. I hated headaches. They always went from the inside through my forehead to my eyes. I always got a headache when I had drunk too much. A headache as I hated. My stomach started to rumble. I began to observe myself carefully. I had the feeling that my hunger decreased a little, and my stomach contracted. I concentrated on my stomach.

I lay on the back, stared at the ceiling and listened to my stomach. This was the situation then in which the headache took a break. Then I felt something like a chill. I pulled the duvet up to the neck and tried to distract myself mentally. At some point, I must probably have fallen asleep. I woke late. It was already after ten. As usual, I went under the shower. This was good. When I take a shower, I inevitably remember my time as a sportsman. At that time, at home, when I was still a child, we would always bathe only on Saturdays. After the sport, however - I started playing volleyball in the school team when I was fourteen -, we were allowed to take a shower. This was always awfully good. I really enjoyed this.

After showering and casual dressing, I went to the kitchen. I sat down at the small plastic table and looked out of the window, lost in thought. I was not hungry at all. The cigarette box, still half-full, caught my eye; I looked away in disgust. If I smoke one now, I thought to myself, I will have lost. I let the thought go on. I imagined smoking a cigarette. I wanted to explore how I felt. I took a cigarette, put it between my lips and left it cold. I took a drag on it and pretended to smoke, even removed the inexistent ash and thoroughly looked at the cigarette. Then I pushed it back into the box – for a possible relapse.

I remained seated and again looked out of the window. It was spring, the blackbirds were trilling, and Dicki came sneaking around the door frame, curved his back like a cat, pushed his hind legs far back and yawned. Coffee, no thanks. The first temptation with the cigarette was overcome, I could more readily renounce the coffee. I dressed and left the flat with the dog. In front of the door, I met my future significant other. She still knew nothing about my starvation diet. She remained aloof and probably wanted to say something, refrained from it, but I asked her:

'Is anything the matter?'

'Haven't you taken a shower, have you been up all night?'

'Humph, I? Quite the contrary, I'm doing thera-peutical fasting.' There was pride in my voice.

'Oh, that's why you stink so much.'

This was more than unpleasant to me.

'You stink like a rotten fish', she capped it all off.

'I must fetch the children from school.'

'OK, and I'll take the dog out.'

At noon I did not go to her and the children. First of all, I had to get rid of the stench again. Even another shower did not help. I had to eat something. But I had no desire at all to eat anything. I remembered that one should 'break' the fasting best of all with fruit. At home I bit into an apple, and I became almost sick. My stomach cramped, I almost vomited. I became a little dizzy, and I lay down on the bed.

Then, in the course of the day, I resumed to eat something, bread, cheese, ham, in the evening spaghetti and a chill rosé. The next day, I did not have so much of an odour any more and visited my new flame.

**Chapter 3**

All that writing is arduous. Months later I am sitting in front of my old laptop again, thinking. I made myself comfortable on the couch in my own room. Opposite of me there is an aquarium, 1,50 metres large, with a black lid and a black base cabinet. Milan, our new hybrid dog, half a dachshund, half a Jack Russel, is lying relaxedly beside me in his full length and is guarding the computer mouse, which, by the way, even works on the couch. The writing is arduous because I want to remember, and at the same time feel that my brain is struggling against it.

And thus it went on:

Three days later, it was the 9th of September, 2010. I had to go to the family doctor again to fetch the lab values, many lab values. The value, that certain value, the creatinine level was at 3.6, the word which I had completely blocked out, there it was again. It was not remotely clear to me then how dramatic this value was. I had fetched the old medical records from the successor of my former family doctor and had browsed them in a hurry. There it was written in black on white, creatinine value 2.8. With that value my then family doctor had sent me to this common-or-garden doctor, this Teuton.

After that, I had not been to the doctor anymore for ten years, until the Indian summer of 2010, because of the life insurance. Dr von Rothenburg, my new family doctor, had examined everything, even with ultrasound. I sat in front of him in his office, and my whole body was trembling. He sent me to the dialysis centre, precisely not just to any specialist. The value 3.6 was enough of an alarm signal, but he had still spoken of other values too, including:

'Your prostate gland is also a little bigger. However, this is not so dramatic.'

Not dramatic? I can think logically, after all. So the other value is dramatic. Thank you, doctor, very sensitive, but now at least I know where I am. The thought struck my head that I am a dialysis patient. I had to swallow, my lips were bursting with dryness, I trembled internally, the blood withdrew from my fingers. I felt how they became colder and colder.

'Here', he said, 'I'll write down the address for you.'

Brutally, with one single jerk, he tore off the uppermost sheet of his yellow block, as large as a beer mat, and stretched it out to me over the table, while he rose. I took the note, stowed it in my purse and gave him my hand. His hand was warm. I left the office like a sleepwalker and slowly made my way home, by foot through the beautiful historic city centre, the good room, as they say here.

I knew every house, every entrance, every shop-window, every historical gable, every church, every cafe, every bar, every restaurant, every street corner. I did not have to look anymore. I had to go to the dialysis centre, to the new one. I still knew the old one, from my time as a student. I had driven taxi, also so-called patient transports. The old-timers, my colleagues then, who went full-time, exactly knew the taxi ranks from which the patient transports were called out, and of course also the times. Then always the same colleagues were standing there. Before I had found out, I had always been surprised why a taxi was waiting all alone on a taxi stand at half past four in the morning, with the engine running, no pub or bar in the whole vicinity, a taxi rank already beyond the town border. No radiocommunication traffic from the headquarters, and then the croaking call into the silence:

'Taxi rank Roxel...'

'Thirteen seven.'

Headquarters:

'Nose, who else. Piusallee 55, patient transport 51 to the dialysis, please help and put down the engine.'

Nose was not his right name; his nose was gigantic, so it was his nickname. Besides, the colleague was so small that he was just barely able to peak above the steering wheel. But he was such a veteran of the taxi business. He was always there where there was clientele, he could virtually smell them. Dialysis transports were longer as a rule, brought good money and were better paid than the normal transports. Besides, the customers were very nice, not drunk, and still gave some tip in addition, although they only had to sign the bill and had to pay no money at all directly. I supposed that many had a bad conscience because they believed to be only a burden for others. I financed almost my whole course of studies with the taxi driving, and so I soon also got to know one address or the other to get hold of dialysis transports.

These were mostly older, very friendly, but for the most part very taciturn people. Thin, yes, I remember, they were all somewhat thin and made an unmotivated impression. There was always a certain stiffness in the taxi. What should we talk about? You do not want to say anything wrong either, put your foot in it, and so we were quiet. Moreover, at that time I dared not really ask them anything. Only the radiocommunication kept interrupting the unnatural, almost morbid silence over and over again. People do not like silence, most people, in any case. I even turned down the radio then. I found it somehow inappropriate to expose these pitiful creatures to pop hits about luck, love and a dream world. Would I be sitting on the kerbside now soon? I felt my shivering in the whole body.

### Chapter 4

Like I said, it was the 9th of September, 2010, a marvellous Indian summer morning, on which I had got the lab values from Dr von Rothenburg. When I left the office, the Indian summer morning seemed unreal to me. The sun shone through the old gabled houses, pushed me, and I felt like on a summer morning at six o'clock in Lisbon.

I often had this association when the sun shone strongly and the air was clear, but still very fresh. Just why Lisbon, Portugal, in 1975 again? It was an especially lighthearted, easy-going, but still tension-loaded time. Midsummer. Backpack, short jeans and sneakers, semester break, revolutionary holidays.

I had spent the night outdoors on many days. There you cannot tighten the blinds. Quiet sunrays touch the eyelids. You wake directly into the day. At that time I used to linger through the historic city centre very early in the morning and to observe how the town slowly woke. The first tramways went, still quite blank. Isolated faces winked through the open windows. Bright idyll, almost in a kitschy way romantical, but true.

The tramway, one of the kind as was known from the television, in San Francisco, a hundred years old, creaky, struggled up the mountain in the direction of the castle. I slowly went behind it. Very quickly it became warm, and I started sweating. I wanted to go completely upwards, let's go the whole hog. I studied sports, among other things, and physical strain always had to do with zest. The first shops opened, small corner shops, with thick wooden doors and wood slats in front of the windows. In front of these there were benches which had, at some time, had some colour. I was greeted as if I went here every morning. The Carnation Revolution was just 1 year old, and even as a stranger you felt the new freedom.

'*Como ela somos livres*', the freedom song of the revolution, could be heard so often that it always sounded in your ears when you looked into these friendly, suntanned faces. The feeling of freedom reached its climax on the mountain of Lisbon. An old grey castle with thick walls and a wide view over the Tejo onto the gigantic bridge which now bore the name of the revolutionary day:

The bridge of the 25th of April – my birthday.

With this feeling I sneaked home through my historic city centre and, with a silent noise, fell into the dark cellar of fear. Dialysis. I am seriously ill. My brain had tried to distract me, to block out reality, the current moment. The impact was all the harder. Come home, I called the dialysis centre, first of all, and a factual female voice reckoned that there would be another free date for making an appointment with Dr Drügeberg on Monday.

Monday, I flipped the calendar, Monday, 13th of September, 2010. Still a whole week.

## Chapter 5

'Are you awake?'

She turned her head to me and expected no answer. 'That you could fall asleep at all! You lay down, dragged the left leg and started to snore. You're a fine one. I pondered at least three to four more hours...'

'I was simply wiped out.'

'I let you be, after all. You've got to come to terms with this, first of all...'

'You see, I'm still alive.'

'You definitely got up seven or eight times tonight. Haven't you noticed this at all, actually?'

'Not really, but I had to go, after all.'

'Why, this could also have to do with the kidneys, couldn't it?'

'You could be right. As you mention this, I remember that the Doc asked about whether I often have to go to the toilet at night. I did not properly answer to this at all. I was not so much aware of it, but now?'

I had already heard from older friends quite a few times that they often had to go out to the toilet at night. This was blamed on age and beer. Yesterday, however, I had drunk no beer or wine at all. Nevertheless, I occasionally had heartburn last night. I had tried simply to block out this thing about the bad kidney values. I seemed to have succeeded in this. Maybe also I did not take it so seriously that I could not survive this.

'Today I will not go to the office.'

'Indeed you had better not; take a rest from the shock for the moment.'

'I am rested enough. Now I am going to take a shower first. Then we'll see what happens. I'll call off the appointments in any case. I can't be doing with them now.'

At breakfast we always sit opposite each other and discuss the day. I had been drinking tea for some time, as that agreed better with me; Beate drank coffee as usual, one or two big pots with very much normal milk. I did not like milk at all, already as a child, in elementary school, and certainly no cocoa from these small bottles which were welded together with aluminium at the top and had such a disgusting skin on top on the cocoa. I had also always drunk my coffee black up to now, especially at the time when I was still smoking, or, as some cynics said, when smoking was still healthy.

I took my two small pills, I still had to halve the one against high blood pressure, and the other was because of the cholesterol. After the breakfast, which was no right one, tea with pills, I went to my study, in which, at that time, there was still no aquarium, but a loft bed, and under it my desk with the computer. I had built the loft bed myself, so massively and solidly that at an earthquake the house could collapse all around, the loft bed would certainly stay. I used this loft bed everytime my wife did not want to endure my snoring any longer and expelled me from the marriage bed.

T-Online, title page, the tabloid of the Internet, full of commercials and insignificant information, but with a column which had not really struck me so much up to now, the column about health. Back pain, today's subject. I moved the cursor to Google and entered 'renal insufficiency'. Already while browsing I felt like in a small veterinary hospital. Kidney failure was and is the main topic concerning sick cats. It took a few pages until I came across the human problem of nephritic illness.

There were many references and links, and it was all too much for me. I wanted to know everything all at once, skimmed through the texts as fast as I could in order to get to the next, with the lasting feeling to miss an important article. At such a surfing speed you cannot understand a lot, but you get carried away. And thus I arrived at cancer and therapeutical fasting. I had already had a positive experience with therapeutical fasting. I had stopped smoking with therapeutical fasting, or better put, I had escaped from this addiction.

Therapeutical fasting has a lot to do with food, or with leaving out food. But fasting is always also about the right food afterwards. Breakfast, finishing the fasting, is a special subject. I became conscious then that you eat nothing the whole night, for the most part, in any case, and the breakfast is basically nothing else but breaking the fasting. If you have arrived at fasting on the Internet, there is not a long way anymore to the concept of nutrition.

This was the moment which changed my life totally. At this moment I did not know yet, but it was a name which I will never again forget in my life:

Helmut Wandmaker.

Besides many other books there was a reference to this small publication titled 'Raw food instead of fire food, true health through natural food (*Rohkost statt Feuerkost, wahre Gesundheit durch natürliche Nahrung*)'. I wrote the title on a small note, shut down the computer and told my wife I would go to town to buy a book. She called after me that I should bring a certain thing. I definitely answered yes and then probably forgot about it again.

It was only just over ten minutes to the city centre. In the bookshop I was almost alone, and behind the info table at the computer there was a young woman with a bun in her hair, wearing round glasses with a black edge. I slipped her the note and looked at her questioningly.

'Good morning'.

'Oh yes, sorry, g'morning. Could you have a look whether you have this in stock?' 'Which publishing company or ISBN?'

'I'm sorry, I forgot.'

'Let's have a look then.'

She strummed on the keyboard and shook her head.

'There is no such book.'

'This is impossible, I only just found it on the Internet.'

'Well, we don't have it in our line. But I'll just look at ....'

I do not know what were all the places where she looked, but after some shaking of the head, redemption came.

'Here, here it is, I found it, we never sold this, it was also never required, but I can order it for you. This will take a few days.'

'A few days? Try to make it faster, please.'

'I'll put "Urgent" on it. Give me your email address, then you will immediately be informed.'

**Chapter 6**

At home I sat down at the computer again. The keyword was and is nutrition, more precisely raw food. There must well be very much more to it than you would generally think. Desperately I looked for Wandmaker and his raw vegetarian food again on the Internet. Surfing can be fun, but if you are afraid, it can become very strenuous. I skimmed the texts like a vulture, always in search of something nutritious, even if I had a strange feeling because I did not exactly know what I was actually looking for. Then again such a term: Baselife.

'Baselife is essentially about the subject "live more consciously, more naturally and more intensely."

It is about raw food, decontamination, fasting, psyche, love and about a comprehensive consciousness in general.'

This is what Bernd Bieder wrote on his homepage. This young man with likable looks is a writer and travel photographer and offers summer camps and fasting walking. Somewhere he had also referred to the book of Wandmaker. I just could not find it now. I am just too stupid, I cannot see the wood for the trees.

Google and simply enter Wandmaker. Quite simply and unerringly. Helmut-wandmaker.de. There it was, not the book, to be sure, but his homepage, including his curriculum vitae. He even founded an endowment. Oh, he passed away in 2007, nearly 94 years old. On account of his heavy illness he dealt with nutrition and wrote three books. He is an honorary citizen of his hometown and received the honourary doctorate from the Ukrainian university. I click on the forum. It was interrupted and should soon function again.

### Chapter 7

Forum. Again a new word which gave me the idea to look for forums. I am no Internet specialist, and Google should help once more. I wrote nutrition and renal insufficiency, thus or similar, into the small box. There were really forums, one in Switzerland: www.symptome.ch. But what should I discuss with them? What do I know, actually, about my illness? What hurt me, actually? What devastated me so much then? Fear. The fear of something uncertain. The fear to die suddenly, but of what. My kidney values were dramatic. I felt silly myself. I would have liked best to cure them immediately without knowing what was wrong, actually. At the bottom of the Google page one was written kidney function. Under www.med4you.at I had found what I probably believed to search, the first important step.

Logic was not really foreign to me, but my logic had certainly taken a break, and it became clear to me that fear is the worst counsellor. I had to proceed logically, and this approach was probably suited for this purpose with the help of this article:

'The function of the kidney. Major tasks: decontaminates by-products, adjusts the body water, adjusts many other materials (e.g., sodium, potassium). In addition every kidney contains approx. 1 million so-called nephrons. … In the nephrons the blood is filtered … namely in a ball made up from minute blood vessels, the glumerulus.

In this, 180! litres of so-called primary urine (first urine) are filtered per day. Except protein and the cells, it contains almost everything which is in the blood. So a lot more than we want to get rid of. Then this primary urine flows through the nephritic tubes (tubuli). Meanwhile the kidney gets some materials from the primary urine, and a lot of water back again… and eliminates other materials, in addition. … Many materials are eliminated in the tubes and then reabsorbed again, or the other way round.

This apparently pointless process allows an exact regularisation of the excretion of a material. Then at the end about 1.5 litres of urine are left per day.'

## Chapter 8

Even if you are not a doctor, and I am certainly not one, it becomes clear, nevertheless, that the kidney keeps the blood clean very cleverly, amends over and over again and takes care that we filter out the materials which strain or even poison our body. What does that mean for me? My kidneys do not filter properly anymore, more and more pollutants remain in the body, until I die of poisoning without really noticing it. I did not have any pain yet. I must ask the doctor some time whether there are any signs. Funnily enough, I do not even look ill at all, and I have also had a good breakfast this morning, two bread rolls with cheese, a five-minute-egg, two cups of coffee, along with the newspaper and the firm will to get some information and not to work. My family doctor had given me the lab values, so that I should take them to the dialysis clinic, but I had neither copied them, nor studied them in detail, only one term had remained in my memory: creatinine. Google: creatinine.

### Chapter 9

What is creatinine? I always exactly want to know everything. Moreover, I had only one day until the appointment at the nephrologist's in the dialysis clinic. So I wanted to be preinformed at least to such an extent that he notices that I know. I did not want by any means to appear silly or unknowing. So back to the Internet.

'Renal insufficiency.'

A certain Private Lecturer Wolfgang Hübl, MD, talks lengthily there and writes:

'For that purpose it is necessary to speak of creatine first. Creatine occurs in the human muscles. It is a material which can store energy and, when required (muscle work), can deliver it again. Approx. 1-2% of the muscular creatine is diminished per day to creatinine.

The creatinine is the by-product of the creatine. The creatinine has – as far as is known – no function, it is a sort of rubbish which is eliminated through the kidney.'

And he writes further:

'Why do we measure creatinine in the blood? Creatinine is eliminated through the kidney. If the kidney does not work properly, then excretion also will not work properly. Then less will be excreted. However, creatinine will be released further from the muscle without reduction. Result: the blood level rises. The creatinine in the blood (more precisely: in the blood liquid) is hence an indicator for the function of the kidney.'

For healthy readers, and so it would have been for me earlier, these explanations are actually unimportant, and they are not perceived in such a way as if you are concerned by it. But I have heard on the radio that one in five men over 60 years old has a renal disease without knowing it. By the way, the word part 'creat' is derived from Greek and means meat. The word creature is indeed more familiar to us. Even if it is laborious for the simple-minded reader to read about even more medical things, I consider it very necessary to recognise that it is not so easy to deduce the right thing from the lab values about creatinine. I also have the impression that quite a lot of doctors do not exactly know a lot about the subject, and specialists partially contradict each other and in my case even only shook their heads when I spoke of my kind of healing attempt. But I will deal with this later. This will even become really exciting.

It is especially important to me that readers do not panic if you immediately run to your doctor and the lab value shows a raised creatinine level. Here Dr Hübl from the Internet helps us again:

'What is to be observed when judging the creatinine level... The creatinine level depends on the muscle mass. Hence, athletic people have higher values than others, men higher ones than women, children different ones from adults and old people. As far as available, the value must thus be compared to the suitable normal values.'

And he writes further:

'A diet rich in meat leads to (somewhat) higher values.'

Here, for the first time, nutrition is referenced by a nephrologist: 'In meat there is, after the cooking, an appreciable amount of creatinine. Under normal circumstances, this will have no determining influence on the creatinine level, in extreme cases it can raise it (bodybuilder with big muscle mass and high meat consumption, and possibly also creatine consumption).'

It is quite evident that you cannot bluntly assign certain morbid effects to the lab values, but precisely in assessing creatinine, you must particularly pay attention, and a detailed consultation with specialists is absolutely necessary. To make this clear, I will let Dr Hübl explain further: 'Creatinine rises only in case of a more intense restriction of the kidney function. The normal filtration amount of the kidney is about 125 ml (= 1/8 litres) per minute. Only if this rate is decreased to about 60-40 ml/min., the creatinine starts to rise in the blood. In between, the damage to the kidney is not recognised. This is also called the area blind to creatinine. Hence, creatinine is not suitable for an early diagnosis of kidney damages.'

Now , however, things are getting still more complicated. Despite this, do not let yourself deter from continuing to follow Dr Hübl, because after all, this is important now in order to understand in which situation I am:

'The amount of the creatinine only makes a limited statement about the extent of the kidney damage. It is, of course, a fact that in connection with a greater kidney damage a higher creatinine level will appear than with a small damage. This is, however, not a strict relationship; a doubled creatinine level does not mean a halved filtration rate. This is due to the fact that, in case of a limited filtration, we can also get rid of creatinine in other ways: The kidney then increasingly eliminates creatinine (secretion); moreover, creatinine is then also eliminated through the bowel. This means that the extent of the kidney damage is underestimated with the creatinine level. However, this is also true vice versa. If our kidney recovers again after a sudden (acute) kidney failure, and the filtration rate increases again, then the creatinine level will hardly sink in the beginning...'

If your family doctor transfers you to the specialist, the nephrologist, you will be assigned the homework to collect your urine for 24 hours. Dr Hübl explains:

'If at the same time you determine the urea (or BUN) in the blood, you are able to calculate the so-called urea-creatinine ratio, which can help to distinguish the different causes of the raised creatinine level.'

If you are in top health, you do not ask yourself why you are healthy, where the health comes from. No, only if things do not work in a normal way anymore, if you are getting worse and worse and you do not know why, then you go to the doctor or chemist, inform yourself and look for causes. Dr Hübl helps us there too: "Which discomfort and signs (symptoms) exist in connection with a raised creatinine level? If you take the creatinine level and the glomerular filtration rate (GFR) as an indicator for the extent of a slowly running (chronic) kidney failure, you can roughly make the following classification:' (end of quotation).

In order not to come up with the chart and statistics at this point, I will describe the symptoms in the order of the course of disease:

The whole problem can start with lack of appetite, tiredness, lack of performance and high blood pressure.

These are phenomena which you blame, first of all, to other causes. I have blamed my professional stress for my general tiredness. Moreover, I am approaching sixty, and so it is probably inevitable that you are not so efficient anymore.

High blood pressure, well, maybe I am not doing enough of physical exercise, and I sometimes get upset more easily, it is not my fault that others are so stupid.

But with a chronic kidney failure, everything becomes just slowly worse. You feel physically weaker and weaker, you lose weight, and it starts to itch. However, this is already a danger signal.

I had not lost weight, though - quite the contrary, even gained some; the evening wine and preferably some sweet food in addition, nougat chocolate etc., did not remain without consequences.

No, what startled me was the itch. During the last weeks I would sit in front of the television and mechanically push my trousers higher up from the socks to the knees and scratch my shins until they were sore and bled.

**Chapter 10**

The day before the first visit at the nephrologist's should change my life radically. I could not anticipate this at this moment yet, but I already had a strange feeling when I saw the book.

'Should I wrap it up as a present for you?'

I must have stared at the young woman with an open mouth and my eyes wide open, horrified. I was not up to such a question. I, only I, wanted to have the book. She shrugged her shoulders, took a small plastic bag and wanted to stow away the book in it.

'No', I shouted excitedly, 'you do not need this, I'll take the book just like that, this will spare the environment', and already stretched out my hand.

'You do want to pay for it, though, don't you?'

I laid eight euros onto the counter, got the book with a receipt and swaggered to the revolving door, uttering the words:

'Thanks, many thanks.'

In the pedestrian zone, I pulled the receipt, which was a little protruding, from the book and flipped it open. Contents. Two pages of table of contents. Was there a register? Right at the end. N.Klm, n, nutrients, nutritional values, sodium, sodium chloride, kidneys. Well. Twelve page references. The first reference to page 25. I searched the page, and while I automatically walked through the pedestrian zone, I skimmed over the page. It was even emphasised in bold type:

'Protein and starch residues thicken and block your fine capillaries in the prostate gland as well as in all other important organs, such as coronary arteries and kidneys.'

There, I thought to myself. But what does that mean now? I will read all this most thoroughly. I shut the book with a snap and directly ran home at a quick pace. On the internet I had found out days before already that Mr Wandmaker's concern was raw food, better put, the consumption of fruit and leaving out all poison materials to clean the body. For three days I had been paying attention to eating as much fruit as possible and drinking no alcohol.

'Did you get what you were looking for?' my wife received me in the floorboard when I unlocked the door to the flat.

'Yes, and I have absolutely no time now.'

'Do you want to go to the office after all?'

'No, I want to read the book, there is more in it about kidneys than I thought. I need absolute quiet now.'

'It's all right, but remember, tomorrow it will be the dialysis clinic, and in one week we'll fly. We'll still have to prepare a few things.'

It was the first time that I had forgotten about a holiday. We had already booked half a year ago. Only for one week, Majorca, a holiday flat in the centre of Palma. Just to get out for a change. We had taken no holiday for about a year already. I really needed a break. And then this diagnosis. For three days already I had drunk no wine, no glass of beer. And now to Majorca? Was this possible at all, to sit in the harbour bar with a glass of water and admire the ships, no iced Canya (beer) with the look into the red evening sun?

**Chapter 11**

It was only half past eleven after all. I ran directly through the flat, then through the kitchen to the terrace. It was pleasantly warm and I browsed through the book by Mr Wandmaker. Next reference, page 38:

'Do you really prefer struggling all your life with some drugs for the treatment of the blood liquid, and in this way perhaps damage your liver and kidneys, and in the end destroy them?'

No, I did not want this at all. I read the whole page from top to bottom. This was rather taken out of context. I flipped the register open again and searched the next page reference under the heading kidneys: page 40 on top:

'... the constant demand to which our adrenal glands are exposed puts the affected persons into those states of disease...'

So I must take more time and read the whole chapter first, or else I will not understand it at all. So I look further for direct findings. Page 44:

'The German Arnold Ehret was a hundred percent advocate of fruit food. He thus overcame his long-lasting heavy renal disease, which 24 doctors could not cure.'

Yes. This was t h e sentence. Now there was no stopping me anymore. My eyes had not yet looked at the end of the sentence when my brain had decided everything. This sentence was like a key experience.

A glimmer of hope?

This was sheer madness.

I felt my heart beat, up to the neck, I was excited, tense, and I clenched my hands into fists.

For me it was certain, I will go this way. Nobody will argue me out of it.

## Chapter 12

I had not noticed at all that my wife was standing behind me.

'What's wrong with you? You're trembling. What's the matter?'

She was afraid, afraid for me. She was really worried about me, while I was only circling around myself.

'I believe I am on the right track. I told you about that Helmut Wandmaker, on the Internet, who was so seriously ill and had changed his food and became healthy again, with fruit.'

'This may well have been so, but it may also have been an isolated case, or what do I know. In any case, you have not starved yet. This is already reassuring.'

'I have not only eaten fruit, but also everything else, just drunk no alcohol and no coffee.'

'Well, it was high time you stopped drinking.'

'I haven't even drunk so much at all, well, a little beer or wine in the evening.'

'Well, you can understate things. It was too much in any case.'

Of course she was right, but who really likes to admit mistakes, especially if you want to continue them because it seems necessary to be able to enjoy your evening. Nobody who drinks no alcohol at all can understand this. But I could not tell her this, after all.

'Here, look what Wandmaker writes here. Here the issue is not his clinical picture, but a healing of kidneys. This is the first time that I read such a thing. Arnold Ehret has gained control of his renal disease only by eating fruit. This is unique.'

'The fact that fruit is healthy is quite clear. I always eat a lot of fruit, and when you drink your wine, I eat my grapes, and I feel well then. I really feel how the energy goes into my brain. And I may not eat oranges in the evening at all, otherwise I cannot even fall asleep and lie awake the whole night. What should we prepare for lunch then?'

I had already read the other lines and had listened to her only with half an ear. Maybe because I had heard it too often already, or because she was right, at least in this point. We never argued, actually, but we discussed very violently for the sake of the matter without hurting each other. Beate was and is the fairest person whom I have ever got to know.

'Fruit.'

'Well, then we won't go shopping. Should be all right to me. I'll still have to do the whole laundry anyway.'

This is her way, not angry, but understanding, responsive to my wishes, somehow positive.

„We should go shopping, nevertheless. To the wholefood market, I want to have a closer look at the fruit bar. Will you come along?'

'Sure, I can do the laundry later still. And I also need milk, washing-up liquid, hand soap and toilet paper, there is hardly anything left of it. Some cold cuts wouldn't be bad either, and the bread is running short; we also have no more yoghurt.'

**Chapter 13**

To me it was clear that today I could call no customer and make appointments. I wanted to read on. In the wholefood market it is like in all other supermarkets. If you enter the shop, you immediately reach the fruit and vegetables department. Why this is so has become clear to me only much later. Now I was standing in front of it, in front of the copious shelves: kiwis, pomegranates, mangos and fruits to which I had not paid so much attention up to now because I did not even know them at all. Neither did I know how you eat them, with bowl or without, or only the stones. It was somehow embarrassing for me to ask somebody and thus to reveal the fact that I did not even know these fruits, which had always been there, but to which I had never resorted. Ap-

45

ples, pears, peaches, bananas, plums, apricots, pine-apples, such things were known to me, and you always took quite at random what just came to your mind or caught your eye. Now I looked in a different way. I wanted to get an overview, and other types of fruits, which I did not know yet, and the apples struck me.

The apples because to me it became clear for the first time how many types were offered here, ten types. This surprised me very much, although I have been making purchases for many years here. I took different apples, a few bananas and figs, ten figs. They cost 59 cents a piece and came from Turkey. I knew figs from Majorca. At that time I had bought one or two at the market to try them. I would never have bought so many earlier on. 5.90 euros, that is indeed a steep price. You already got two schnitzels for it. My wife had looked after the other things, and one hour later we were sitting in the kitchen again, having lunch. Beate took some slices of bread with salami and cheese and put a glass of sour gherkins on the table for herself. I took one fig after the other, cut them in the middle and scraped them clean with a teaspoon as you scrape kiwis. After the eighth fig I was exhausted.

'You are not quite full already, are you?' she asked me.

'Somehow yes. I cannot eat any more figs, and I don't fancy apples either. Somehow I am quite full, but somehow I am not. I'm going to doss down for a short while.'

I took my Wandmaker and disappeared into my room. Thirst drove me into the kitchen two more times that evening. I completely missed the television programme, the news, some film and the news of the day, which I otherwise always watched. Wandmaker had put me under his spell.

## Chapter 14

20th of September, 2010. Monday, half past nine, and we were sitting by gate 13 in the airport. We had one more hour of time. In my dark red canvas bag from the wholefood market there were different apples, two clementines, which can be peeled better than oranges, and two bananas. I had provided for the trip to Majorca.

'I would like to drink a coffee', Beate whispered, bending over to me.

'Well, let's go. However, I would only like a glass of water. Go ahead and look for a place for us, I'll go to the bar. Would you want anything else?'

'Maybe a bread roll, with cheese.'

Thus I had already changed. Earlier, before we both drove somewhere, I had always prepared bread roll, and amply, best with liverwurst and mustard and with salami, and of course with cut cheese. This does not always immediately smudge so much. For bread rolls are always crushed on the way. Today I had provided for nothing, as far as the bread rolls were concerned, in any case, but for fruit, for her and for me. Since very recently there were only dishes on order in the airplane, for all others sandwiches. 'Cheese or sausage?' I heard the stewardess call, already quite far behind me. Most people took sausage. When she was then standing in front of us, I shook my head, Beate said:

'Cheese'.

'I'll take one with cheese after all', I added. Beate smiled, and I handed over my sandwich to her as well.

'You must still become big and strong', I grinned at her.

'Look who's talking', she retorted. I reached into my canvas bag and rummaged around for an apple.

Then the second carriage came through the middle course. Beate took a coffee again, I an orange juice.

After the landing everything was, actually, as usual, and we went to Palma by taxi. The holiday flat was in the middle of the centre in a very narrow lane in the first floor. The landlord was adjusted to Germans and spoke German fluently. Then in the flat, after introducing us to the use of the remote control of the satellite TV, he wanted to explain to us the cooker and the oven. At that point, however, I automatically waved my hand and said self-confidently:

'We do not cook'.

'Ah, you will go out for a meal; I can recommend you some good restaurants in the town.'

'That is very nice of you', I interrupted him as politely as possible.

'But we know Palma very well, we've already come on the island for nearly 20 years. We love Palma.'

This seemed to have excused my interruption again.


## Chapter 15

We lingered through the lanes, stopped in front of the same Jugendstil houses as we used to, admired anew the known ornaments, the arcs and gables. We had to find out with regret that the small Café de Isla had closed down, still much worse, it was emptied. Maybe they are just doing reconstructions, we both thought at the same time and came to an agreement by looks.

'I slowly get hungry', said Beate.

On holidays I always liked to be the chef, or we went to eat a little, preferably pizza at an Italian restaurant on the Plaza mayor right in the centre. This place was *the* place in Palma. Here one of many markets takes place, there were always pantomimes which moved atypically for a few cents and in particular attracted children. The Christmas fair is always here too, and when nothing is going on, every cafe is open and has put up all chairs and solar decks almost up to the middle of the place. Street musicians alternated, and it was always an experience just to sit there and to observe the people while having a glass of wine.

The thought of the wine was not only enticing, but virtually tantalising. A cool rosé simply belonged with it all. How should it work without it? The first thought was not to go at all to the Plaza mayor, as Germans to the Italian restaurant in Spain. However, I did not want to do this to Beate either. She felt so fine there, in distant, but usual surroundings, an absolutely relaxed atmosphere, of which you always only dreamt at home and longed for going there again. So I will just drink no wine, water is also healthier after all, and I must simply try it out once.

'Okay', I said and nodded.

'To our Italian restaurant?' she asked and already turned around in the direction to the Plaza mayor. This was, of course, only a rhetorical question, and I would have had to evoke something powerful to make an alternative literally palatable. The waiter recognised us again and offered us our regular seat, which was still free by chance. It was late afternoon already, and the sun shone like at home in midsummer. It was pleasant under the big summer tarpaulins, but the air was dry and a little dusty. There must have been no rain for a long time, I thought and looked around. It is a low season, and the members of the infamous skittles clubs had meanwhile got a good night's sleep and pervaded Palma. At some time they all got stuck at this place. The beaming sun, a lot of cafés and restaurants, no cars, and German was spoken, and if you did not especially order Spanish beer, there was German one, and not only one type.

We were surrounded by some older couples and groups, who remarkably quietly raised their glasses to each other. Ice-cold Pilsner, and what is more, cleanly tapped.

'To drink?'

I turned back to the table. The waiter laid the menu on the wooden table for my wife and then for me and looked directly into my eyes.

'A moment, *por favor*'.

'I'll have a glass of water, *con gaz*', Beate bridged my pause for reflexion.

'So will I, however still.'

She looked questioningly and yet quite admiringly at me.

'You really want to go through with it', she stated.

'Yes, and you know me. I have drunk no alcohol as a child and was also content and happy."

Did I only fool myself now, and did I look for serious strategies to strengthen my will to drink water? We both skimmed through the menu. My counterpart seemed to have found something fast.

'I don't know what I should take', I said, and then she:

'Just take a salad, there is a big choice.'

I had skimmed through the page with the salad offers already several times, but I wanted neither crunchy chicken or turkey filets, sardines or tuna, but just plain salad. The waiter came back and brought us the water. My wife took half a chicken with chips and salad.

'I would like only a salad without fish and meat', I said in a strainedly self-confident manner.

'Which dressing?'

'Nothing, and also no salt and pepper, *por favor*.'
'*Vale,* I'll bring this you separately with pleasure.'

And thus it happened. To the salad plate he put the small decanters with oil, vinegar and the duo of salt and pepper shakers in addition. I spiked a salad sheet on the fork and hoped that afterwards the tomato would taste better. Dark balsamic vinegar used to bring me the taste, and now it all tasted unsavoury and like water, and the tomato tasted like the iceberg lettuce. And I was hungry. For nearly two days I had only eaten fruit, and actually I would have had to devour the salad. I had not even the desire to chew the salad properly, but only to devour it as quickly as possible just to get something into my stomach at all. I also did not want to return it. It was not the salad's and the waiter's fault, after all. Both just looked the same as in the last holiday. I have worked temporarily as a waiter when I was a schoolboy, and even today I have a rotten feeling when I return something. It is somehow embarrassing for me, even if I were in the right.

'I'll never order such a salad again. I'll spend no more money on it,' I quietly groaned to myself. Beate shrugged her shoulders. My mood had hit rock bottom. We paid, friendly and with tip, as usual, and went in silence through the narrow lanes of Palma.

'Have a look, this looks good,' shouted Beate and pointed at a small shelf with fresh, luminous oranges, in between, cleverly distributed, some brilliant lemons, even with pale green small leaves on them. The shelf was so overloaded that you almost did not perceive the entrance at all.

'Have a close look,' I said. 'I know the shop. When we were here with the children last time, our potential daughter-in-law had selected something for her mother here, because they have here the speciality of Majorca, the sharp sausage of the black pig, you remember?'

'Yes, now I see it too. I was properly blinded by the oranges because I was looking for something tasty for you,' she answered.

'They sell no fruit at all, but only sausage, ham and olive oil.'

Since this especially striking lure system, we were sensitised and found examples of this advertising method by the dozen. Even the hotdog booth promoted fresh oranges; whether food stores, bakers, ice-cream parlours, cafés, and even butchers attracted the attention of the passers-by to themselves, or to their shops, by means of fresh fruit. The buffets in Chinese restaurants, the shelves in Italian ones or the Tapas in Spanish ones, everything was garnished with colorfully arranged fruit. Only in a supermarket we could buy what was up to then only allowed to be admired in the shop windows: Fruit.

We stocked up so amply on mangos, oranges, kiwis, nectarines, bananas and melons that we needed two carrier bags to transport everything into our holiday apartment.

## Chapter 16

The third pure fruit-only day was the first entire day of our holidays on Majorca. For breakfast I peeled off two big juicy mangos. They were hard to peel, they were so juicy. I licked the thick cores like chicken's clubs, and my hands dripped with the juice, and my mouth was smudged all around. Beate, who enjoyed her coffee as usual, only shook her head.

'I will not only wash myself immediately, but I must even still take a shower, don't worry', I babbled to her with my mouth filled.

'You sorely need this too, because you stink like an elk', she grumbled back.

'No, you mean like a rotten fish!' I returned.

'Exactly, just like when you did this fasting.'

„Therapeutical fasting, my dear, therapeutical fasting. That way, however, I escaped from puffing at that time. As soon as you get back to eating normally then, the smell leaves again.'

'Then I am curious how this will go on. Aren't you really hungry at all?' she asked.

'No, not really. I had even decided to eat even more fruit after the mangos, but this does not work at all. I don't get any more in. Also no need to. And I felt fit as a fiddle. Let's hang out and do something great!'

A small hired car is worth its weight in gold on Majorca. Thus you can explore the whole island and visit small towns which are not flooded by the masses. In three to four places there is always a market on the island, if not in Palma, then in Pollensa, if not there, then in Deya or Valdemosa. In the German-language weekly magazine, called the *'Mallorca-Magazin'* or simply MM, these and other dates are described in detail and regularly.

Whoever knows Mediterranean weekly markets does not need any raving on about them. Whoever is eager to buy fresh fruits, however, can almost become mad. You may try not only the bright or dark grapes, the oranges are squeezed directly in front of the customer. Your mouth is watering. This or similar must be how paradise felt.

As an inhabitant of a Christian-influenced Europe I know, of course, that Adam and Eva lived only on fruits, agriculture and cattle breeding were, after all, the punishments – 'in the sweat of thy face' - after the expulsion from paradise. There are anthropologists who agree with the Old Testament in this point and are convinced that people were fruit eaters for millions of years. Also I slowly have the feeling that with healthy teeth you can bite hard into an apple, but you have no sabre-teeth like a tiger to tear muscles off the bones.

'I ask myself,' I said, addressing Beate, who stood in front of a long table with hand-worked jewellery:

'Why it was just an apple or fruit tree in paradise, and a tree of knowledge about good and evil at that?'

'How are you getting at that subject right now?' she asked, surprised.

'For me this is a contradiction. Fruit seems to be the healthiest food, and there was nothing else in paradise, and the fruits which looked especially tasty and enticing, you might not eat, and if you did, you knew more than before. I am very glad that I know more today than two weeks ago. And, I feel better than ever before at that. And moreover, if I know what is good and evil, I can still decide whether I want the good or evil, especially as I am convinced that evil does not exist at all. This is only an abstract word which exists in itself only in language, a pure human invention. Though there are evil people, and plenty of them, but evil in itself does not exist.'

While Beate had listened, she disagreed, and for her, God also existed.

**Chapter 17**

It was quite late afternoon when we entered our holiday apartment again. In my whole life I have never dragged as much fruit in bags as on this day. The fruit bowls were not sufficient, we also took the salad bowls and soup plates and distributed them on the tables and the shelves of the fitted kitchen. It looked intoxicatingly colorful. A little exhausted, I lay down on the sofa, while Beate prepared a coffee for herself. I closed my eyes. I was tired, and yet could not fall asleep. I was tired, and I had got used for a long time to doss down at noon.

But lately I was also tired in the morning, I who was actually an early bird. For some weeks, Beate had woken me up in the morning. And if I think about it properly, I had always been quite exhausted lately. I had blamed this on my professional strain. But since I knew about my catastrophic kidney values, I could imagine very well that this was associated with them. My stomach was rumbling, and I got hungry. Without opening my eyes, I quietly said:

'I believe I slowly get really hungry. This already almost hurts. Only I absolutely don't fancy any fruit.'

Beate stirred in her big coffee pot and sat down to me.

'You should eat something real again. Your stench has already decreased, though', she said in a very low voice, rather to herself than to me.

'However,' she continued, 'just speaking of it: Has it actually struck you that you do not snore anymore since you stopped drinking beer? And your dropouts are also gone. I always was quite afraid you would stop breathing. This is much better anyway than before. But I have always said this to you, about the alcohol. You did not want to admit it.'

'What do you think how much I would like to drink a freshly tapped Pilsner now – did I say one? No, no, I won't do that, don't worry, and I'm firmly persuaded I would get sick to my stomach in the current situation.'

'So don't do this, please. The day is still long, we can simply go out somewhere for dinner afterwards?'

Inevitably, I had to think of the salad. My stomach seemed to turn round even further at the thought.

'No,' I said determinedly, 'just not to any restaurant. You know what, we'll go to the next supermarket, you remember, under the *Plaza mayor*. This is very near, and we'll get a package of spaghetti with some tomato sauce. This would be enough for me. Preferably even a little minced meat. Or rather not. For minced meat it is somehow too hot here, who knows whether this is still good. I don't trust the

Spaniards so much there. And neither do I want to poison us.'

Less than two hours later we were standing in front of the cooker and frowned.

'Do you remember what the landlord had said how you turn on the cooker?' I asked into the open.

'No,' she sighed, 'I had thought you wanted to cook nothing at all.'

I began to fumble for all buttons, turned where you could turn, sometimes to the left, sometimes to the right, and pulled every lever. Then I opened the oven door, and the operating instructions slid in front of my feet. Not turning, not pulling, pushing was the solution. Really, the big rear burner became red. I put a pot on it and got a bottle with a litre of mineral water from the cupboard. With the tap water you could take a shower at most, and being experienced in Majorca, we knew our stuff.

'So, Beate, if now I already sin, however, I renounce salt, I have sworn this to myself. OK?'

She only shrugged her shoulders and nodded. I had told her about the knowledge about salt immediately when I surfed on the Internet a few days ago at home and had come across the diseased cats. The cat food is much too salty, and that was one reason among others why especially domestic cats suffered so strikingly often from kidney failure. But people also have this problem. It was explained by the fact that in the evolution, people hardly approached salt over millions of years, although the body needs salt. And because there was so little salt, the body has already gathered it quite diligently and hoarded it, namely in the kidney. In former times people could not take up too much salt at all.

Today, in contrast, everything is virtually over-salted, and in the ready-made food, salt is included excessively. Now you could suppose that the kidney delivers the excessive salt again. It does not, how-ever. It throws everything else out, just not the salt. So the versatile and extremely complex job of the kidney is disturbed, right up to kidney failure. Mod-ern people take in too much salt, and I had read somewhere that one out of five sixty-year-old men in Germany has a kidney disease without knowing it. The tomato sauce was so salty that you would not really have had to tilt any more salt into the noodle water.

With ravenous hunger I had devoured the spa-ghetti. My stomach arched, and there was only a small step to the sofa. I had to lie down.

When I woke again, it was quite dark outdoors. A yellowish street lantern made the contours of the pieces of furniture a little visible. I dragged myself on into the bedroom, and what did I hear – my wife was snoring. Tomorrow I will tell her this, I thought to myself and fell asleep.

**Chapter 18**

In my dream I must have been taken to a sauna which was closed from the outside, so much was I drenched in sweat when I woke up. My shirt was soaking wet, and I was convulsed with pain. Slowly I felt where the pain came from. It was my stomach. There was pressing, there was dragging, there was pinching, all at the same time. I curled up, turned onto my belly and pulled up my knees so close to myself that my belly hung in the air. I felt a relief and remembered pictures of pregnant women who also relieved themselves in this way. Then I slowly crept from the bed. Beate did not snore anymore.

Below on the ground the light of the street lantern took pains going through a narrow slit. This had to be the door. I went out over the small hall through the sitting room to the open kitchen. I searched for the mineral water. Water is supposed to work miracles with poisoning, after all. Had I poisoned myself? What had I eaten?

Through the kitchen window the orange-yellowish street lantern unfolded its full medieval splendour, and I could see the kitchen unit with the cooker in the middle. The bulky 5-litre bottle with drinking water, which we also used for brushing our teeth, was standing in the sink. A gigantic gulp, and the water was running along the corners of my mouth onto my vest. I had a pleasant feeling. My stomach gurgled and rumbled. I took off my vest and crept back into bed. I sat down with a straight back to the pillow and waited.

Spaghetti, no, I'll never eat them again. But they could not have been poisoned after all. It was the noodles themselves which tormented me so much. I am also not quite clear in my head. How can I eat only fruit for nearly four days and then fill up my stomach so much at once. More out of proportion was not possible. Nevertheless, I did not reproach anything to me. I must and want to learn from it. Are noodles really so bad, or was it rather due to the fact that I changed too massively from the fruit back to the usual food?

What are noodles, actually? Semolina without egg. Thus it is always written on the package. But what is semolina? Strange, why don't I actually know this? And why did I have this ache in my stomach, why could I not digest this actually normal serving just as much as before? Did I not only have a kidney disease? Did I have a peptic ulcer and even stomach cancer?

Now this is enough, I thought to myself. I do not want to go crazy now. And somehow I dropped off then.

### Chapter 19

It is crazy, though – you eat spaghetti with all possible and impossible sauces with pleasure your whole life long, and you do not know at all what you are taking in there. But everybody I know likes to eat noodles. The children preferably the original with tomato sauce, Italian spices and Parmesan cheese, everything in a package.

This cannot really be bad if everybody eats it and even competitive athletes, because of the calories. I would not be me if I did not examine this more closely. My first step is: Wikipedia. Actually, everybody can look up or click this, and I can only advise to do this. Since just because many people do something, that does not mean by a long shot that it is reasonable per se. To save you the trouble at this point, we will just go to Wikipedia together:

'The hard wheat (Triticum durum) is, after soft wheat (Triticum aestivum), the economically most important kind of wheat. Cultivation occurs, as a rule, as a summer grain. ...

The flour is especially rich in glue [3], the elastic dough won from it [1] is particularly suited to the production of pasta....'

Now I am interested in the concept 'rich in glue':

Gluten (from lat. gluten = 'glue'); synonyms: Glue, glue protein) is a collective term for a material mixture of proteins which occurs in the seed of varieties of grain.

With water added to the flour, it is the gluten which forms a rubber-like, elastic mass in pasting. It has a central importance for the baking qualities of flour. Components of the gluten can lead to celiac disease in people with a corresponding disposition, an inflammatory disease of the intestinal mucous membrane with far-reaching health consequences.'

Whether by chance or consciously, I suddenly found myself on the page carbohydrates – Wikipedia. What I read there was an eye-opener to me. This had never become as clear to me as at the moment I read this:

'Because many saccharides show the gross formula $Cn(H_2O)m$, it was falsely thought that they are hydrates of the carbon, which is why Carl Schmidt coined the concept of carbohydrate in 1844, which is used to this day.' In plain English this means if you leave all chemical delicacies aside, carbohydrates are sugar, the name is wrong and confusing.

This is why bread also tastes mawkishly if you chew it for a longer time. All grain products consist more or less of sugar, including noodles.

'I was already worried so much. Where have you been?'

'I'm sorry, I would certainly have laid a slip of paper for you on the table, but I could not anticipate that I would need so much time. I was just around the corner in an Internet cafe and printed out something for me . It took so long until the computer guy understood what I actually wanted.'

I read out my printout from Wikipedia to her.

'For that you would not have had to go on the internet. I could also have told you this. You know the daughter of the cousin of my mother. She had this allergy. She would almost have died of it. She does not eat any normal bread anymore at all and bakes her own.'

'This had never become so clear to me that noodles, like bread, are made of wheat or grain. Wandmaker also wrote something about it.'

I had not perused the book by a long shot – Majorca is still so diverse and thrilling, even after 20 years of holidays. But I had the book either always in the pocket or lie on the table, always ready to look into it in every spare minute.

'Page 19. Bread is the material of death. This is the heading. I don't want to read out everything to you, just this here:

"A main problem of the bread and grain food is based on the fact that the damages appear only late and are very hard to cure then. Except for frequent catarrhs, colds, mucious obstructions, beginning stiffening, rheumatic muscle pain, stomach trouble – for example, by heartburn and acid regurgitation – nothing is noticed for the time being."

Stomach trouble, I had that tonight, but don't ask. I had never experienced such a thing till then, except when I had come back from Portugal, and out of so much pain I had gone from the railway station directly to the hospital by taxi, because then I had thought I had poisoned myself. But it was a gastritis together with a grumbling appendix.

It was such a feeling that I also had tonight, only in addition, I had a handball-sized iron ball in my stomach. I can only tell you one thing: I am done with noodles and bread. And today I'm going to eat nothing at all anymore. I'll remain with my clear water. This has been very good for me, by the way.'

'However, please don't exaggerate. I believe you have already lost weight.'

'I also believe this. I have really strapped my leather belt, my favorite belt for over 15 years, more narrowly by one hole this morning . And I feel lighter. What are we going to venture today?'

**Chapter 20**

After a small drive we had arrived in Sa Rapita and stopped by the steep coast. Here the sea always smashes against the stony coast, even if it is not very windy. It is overwhelming over and over again to look at the open sea, to know that over there lies Africa, simply to let your thoughts fly freely, to dream and to enjoy the tranquillity of nature. I had flipped my little book open and had looked for a certain place which I had already flipped open at home when I looked under the term kidneys.

On page 25 the term already appeared.

'Listen what's written here. Only one sentence please. Are you listening?'

'Of course.'

'Text, text and then:

'Grain and sugar slime. Protein and starch residues thicken and block your fine capillaries in the prostate gland as well as in all other important organs, such as coronary arteries and kidneys.'

Here it is written again, the kidneys are always affected.'

We still discussed about that, as usual, for a very long time, and we liked to go through the scenery by car without any hurry and conversed incessantly, and that since we had met for the first time. If you talk a lot with your partner, you develop. You always consider your own thoughts to be right, although they can be wrong. An honest objection, a question or also some criticism is very helpful there, even though or even just because it can be painful.

The famous alternative pedagogue Helmut von Hentig is reported to have once said that in life you should always assume that the other person could also be right. Then there would also be no war, he believed. But it is so difficult to change your own view, maybe even to have to abandon it and to recognise that you are simply wrong in this or that respect.

Why is this so difficult? On one hand, you are always somehow sure of yourself. On the other hand, you are hard pushed to concede something to someone else, to admit that you are wrong yourself. You are ashamed. What is, however, also true over and over again, is this: You cannot properly imagine the other possibility at all because it was always like that, because everybody else also does it like that or thinks in such a way, because it even is written in the Bible. I took the school-leaving exam in an episcopal school, and many contradictions struck me even then, but now it is about something so natural that first of all you have to digest this in the literal sense.

Give us today our daily bread, etc., that's how it says in the Lord's Prayer. And now I must realise that here historical ignorance leads mankind into disease with the highest sanctification. Especially on Sundays we always had bread rolls. For school our mother would always wrap us sandwiches with cheese and sausage, preferably liverwurst. And the French with their crunchy baguette along with cheese, in addition a tart fresh wine. This should all be wrong? Poison us? If this is so, I must change not only any habit I had come to love, but somehow my whole life, and at the age of 58 years.

And, nevertheless, I have succeeded in doing something which I used to consider impossible. I have now lived only on fruit and mineral water for 4 days.

Then came the fiasco with the noodles. When I thought of this night, I felt the pain again. Had my body adjusted so fast? I could hardly believe this. Had I lacked something, during these 4 days? Yes. If I am honest with myself, yes. Even if I have fought with all strength against it, I would have awfully liked to drink a fresh cold beer, and a chill Rosé with the salad. Why have I not bent, nevertheless, and have become weak? I was afraid and continue to be.

Genuine fear is stronger than will or habit. My kidney values are dramatic. After the week in Majorca, I will have to go to the specialist, to the nephrologist. I check with the fingers. In nine days I am going to have the appointment with Dr Fry in the dialysis clinic in the hospital. Another three days of Majorca, the sun, sea, beach and walks through quiet villages and dunes.

## Chapter 21

We had gone on and were now sitting in a fantastically situated café on a raised terrace with a look at the picturesque harbour of Cala Figueira. A postcard of this place of the island could not even be as fascinating as this look. Whoever once sat here and was open for this idyl will come here over and over again. Here you can breathe deeply in the most true sense of the word. It was a low season after all. This could immediately be recognised by the audience: Retirees or families with small children who were not school-age yet, racing cyclists and skittle clubs.

A couple of retirees was sitting in front of us. Both overweight. She enjoyed herself in a thick piece of cake, and in front of him and his round belly there was a big beer mug. One strong gulp had sufficed, and the glass was half-empty.

'If I drank a beer now, I believe I would have to puke', I said to Beate, whose look I caught from the belly of the man.

'Do you still have an ache in your stomach?" she asked.

'No, it's all but gone, and neither am I hungry at all. I'll remain with the water – without gas. You can order what you want, as far as I'm concerned. You would certainly like to eat something, as I can tell by looking at you.'

She nodded and said, 'I must honestly admit this to you. I'm starving to death. I did not want to eat in front of you, you understand?'

'Don't worry about that. That doesn't bother me at all. There is surely some good fish here.'

While I meant this honestly, I had a strange feeling. On one hand, I wanted to be consistent and was also genuinely afraid of having to go to dialysis, on the other hand I know how such a Pilsner tastes, and a pizza with tuna, onions and capers – my brain was rotating in all directions at the same time.

Pizza, that is, after all, also dough, flour and gluten, starch garbage as it was written in the book. I

could eat pizza every day, alternately with an escalope Gipsy style and an espresso afterwards.

I looked down along the rock to the light blue,
slightly turquoise sea. A sailing boat left the harbour
with a quiet engine. The other guests also turned
round. We gazed after the boat as it hoisted the sails
and became smaller and smaller, and then disappeared on the horizon.

Gulls came and screeched. A fishing cutter approached the harbour. The waiter brought the fish,
salad and croquettes to my wife. I did not fancy fish
so much at all. More likely fried fish in the market
with tarter sauce. The smell which went out from
the fish plate was deafening, salty spicy. I felt the
saliva in my mouth collecting. 'Maybe you should not
be so strict with yourself,' said Beate, caringly.

'I have now hung on three days and made a mistake. This mistake was more than instructive. It
made painfully clear to me that I am going the right
way. I want to become healthy again. You know, I
read it out to you, that Professor Ehret also made it,
after 24 doctors could not help him. I have eaten
from the tree of knowledge, and that was a good
thing and not evil or bad. That is so strange anyway.
In paradise there were only fruits to eat, and the
tree of knowledge was an apple tree. Especially in
apples there is virtually everything which people
need to live, and just from that tree Adam and Eve
were supposed to eat nothing. According to the Old
Testament, people actually must have been fruit

eaters by nature. Only when they left paradise, they had to till their fields in the sweat of their faces. This perplexes me very much. Agriculture, baking and bread do not come from paradise, but are a punishment, and that every day. So I must think about it once more in rest.'

I had got quite properly excited.

'You can think what you want, but I believe in God.'

'I wouldn't like to speak of that with you now at all. I would like to enjoy this here now and recover. In a few days we will be at home again. It is allegedly getting cold, and I'll have to go to the doc.'

'You are right, it is nice here over and over again, but don't be too strict with you, so it will not backfire. I worry about you. You must eat something once again.'

I watched her eating and was surprised that I felt good eating nothing.

## Chapter 22

The cells of our human body store sunlight. If you go along on the Mediterranean island in the harbour in Palma, you feel how good the sun is for you. Whether it is about the famous vitamin D or the movement in itself, all doctors tell you over and over again to go to the fresh air a lot, to stock up on some sunshine. However, unfortunately, we cannot take up this light directly from the sun. For that we need living herbal food to be able to store light in our cells and to renew with it their liveliness.

People must eat plants, so fruit, salad and vegetables, otherwise it just will not work. The amount of the light storage in our body cells decides on illness or healing. Thus or similar you can read it in many health journals.

Go for a walk in the sun, you can also do this at home, in Germany, even in winter, and it costs nothing. It is not only good, it is also beneficial. It really helps. Only, why do people not do it? Or rather, not enough.

You also see them sitting here in the harbour, in the cafés, on deck chairs, on their yachts worth millions, and almost everybody too fat. After we were back in the flat from Cala Figueira yesterday, I was not hungry at all. I did not even want to eat an apple or a kiwi, nothing. My wife was already properly worried. I knew this feeling from fasting.

There comes the point when you are not hungry anymore. I was only interested in reading on. I went to bed early to go for an extensive walk the next morning and to buy myself vitamin C. Whoever followed me up to this point will ask themselves, of course, why now vitamin C as well if he has already been taking in only fresh fruit for days? I cannot check scientifically what Helmut Wandmaker writes, but he also does not require this. He only always says you should simply try for yourself. Besides, vitamin C is something special. He writes on page 131:

'For decades, his colleagues insinuated that with the vitamin C, Pauling only produced kidney stones and expensive urine. The American biochemist was able to produce the evidence towards his critics that 95 percent of the additional vitamin C remain in the body and only 15 percent are eliminated by way of the urine. Thus the organism disposes of an extensive vitamin C depot, and no kidney stones will be formed. On the contrary – the function of the kidneys improves considerably after the supply of vitamin C.'

This is why I wanted to go to bed early to buy myself vitamin C from the chemist's shop immediately. In my zeal I did not have the Spanish island clock in my head anymore. All shops, the chemist's shops as well, were still closed, except the cafés. So I used the compulsive break and lingered to the harbour. The harbour is several kilometres long, and opposite is the big six-lane road at which the cafés, restaurants and boutiques line up. Farmacia, the green lamp flashes, a chemist's shop has just been opened. I did not have to explain a lot, but saw the little plastic roles known to me in yellow or orange, vitamin C effervescent tablets.

I immediately took two, an orange one and a yellow one. In the harbour there were several cafés, but one quite near the water and the boats. Some couples had made themselves at home and had an extensive breakfast with croissants and white coffee and boiled eggs.

This looked all very appetizing, but I was not interested in it. When, however, I ordered only one bottle of water without gas and let two vitamin C tablets fall into the glass, I felt their sympathetic looks.

**Chapter 23**

Another two days, I thought, while I let go my eyes over the smooth water, past the small Llauts, the fishing boats of the locals, the sailing yachts becoming greater and greater up to the horizon at the end of the far-reaching harbour of Palma. Another two days to the departure – to the hard reality. I had my camera with me, a small digital camera, and I took a photo of my view to the left, then on and on to the right, and always a click, until I suddenly looked into the face of a guest, who threw me a blink of an eye. This was not really my intention, and it was embarrassing for me. I smiled back and shouted:

'I just wanted to record the panorama, for home, then I will be able to remember exactly my seat here.'

'I did not think you were a spy,' he laughed back.

'Do you also have such headaches? I cannot tell you at all what goes off in my head. No aspirin helps either. There is only one help, a few small glasses of beer. You should resume with what you have stopped with in the evening. You just have to go through it. But the sea breeze is good. These effervescent tablets only make you feel bad. And soon it will also be noon. I must hang on till lunch, then I am always better again when I have something in my stomach. The French rave about champagne in the morning when you have a hangover, but of that I get heartburn in addition. That's why at noon I only drink dry, mild white wine, preferably from Baden. I can only recommend it.'

He turned round jerkily, a friend had knocked him hard on the left shoulder from behind. I did not do the babbling welcoming ceremonial to myself anymore. I paid and left the café without saying goodbye. My neighbour on the right had forgotten me again a long time ago.

I was only too aware of the fact that the general illness of the German residents in Majorca was the alcohol abuse. The apparent paradise, rich and vegetating in abundance, only small talk, golf and parties in order not to feel the desolate boredom in your own brain. I have no buried envy. I do not know envy in itself at all. I am rather the one who is glad for others when they achieve something, are happy and contented. I feel a subliminal compassion or even disdain for such creatures that Chekhov once called summer visitors of this earth who are actually super-fluous. I think more of thinking over the tax system. This quality of life with which I had just been confronted was and is only an apparent quality of life. I am convinced that such people recognise the value of their own lives only by way of a hint.

As banal as it sounds, but lifetime is simply limited. In such contacts, I feel an unrestrained arrogance over and over again, an arrogance without understandable reason. This self-overestimation seems to me almost quite natural, as if it was established in our genes. The so-called modern, educated person knows that cigarettes and alcohol are life-menacingly toxic. Nevertheless they smoke and drink, virtually without rhyme or reason. Even the knowledge about lung cancer, smoker's legs and the most agonising death by suffocation does not deter. The self-overestimation can be a reason why the individual person thinks that all these illnesses always concern only the others. The life of a smoker is always an ordeal.

As a youngster, the individual person is especially subject to a social pressure to which you give way fast because you would not like to be excluded from the group, i. e. would like to be part of it, which is, after all, just all too human. Here already the suffering begins for everybody, psychically and health-wise. This natural weakness of the youth is brutally exploited by adults who earn on the production and distribution of the tobacco.

Besides, however, the fateful thing is that this 'youthful folly' is addictive. Even as an adult you have heavy fights with yourself to stop smoking. The suffering goes on. And it costs a lot of money, not only your own, but it also reaches into the wealth of the society. Whoever cannot escape from smoking must keep on suffering, healthwise anyway.

There is no exception, but at most self-deception, partly by self-overestimation. Also whoever wants to stop and does not make it suffers, if they are honest with themselves. They are, in any case, always complicit in that youngsters take them as role models and fall into this addiction trap. Moreover, smokers stink. The best perfume will not be of any use there.

People breathe incessantly the whole life long, from the first gasp to the last one, day and night in every second, they may never stop, otherwise they will die after a few minutes. If such a state occurs, for example, by an accident, and the person can be revived, their brain will very often not be fully functioning anymore, after a few minutes already, mind you.

We people always, always, always need air, fresh air. Fresh air is existential. Just think of the term smoke poisoning. I had stopped smoking because children had stepped into my direct life. I did therapeutical fasting. When you are fasting, you cannot smoke. You would feel sick immediately. Whoever wants to eat a healthy diet must start with not smoking, escape from this drug which poisons the whole body and penetrates into every cell, into every skin cell, every muscle cell etc.

Only after fifteen years of non-smoking, this is what experts write, the risk of a cardiac infarction has sunk to the level of a non-smoker. Then the danger to fall ill with diabetes has clearly decreased as well, because the cholesterol level is lower and the kidneys work better.

I was so much lost in thought that I had run past the front door of our holiday apartment. At the next crossroad I noticed my mistake and went back.

## Chapter 24

'The day after tomorrow we will already fly back again,' I said.

'Should we drive our loop road again tomorrow, as usual, on the day before departure?' She nodded, and by looking at her, you could tell her joy about going through the central destinations of the last few days once again.

'That does not mean, however, that we will venture nothing today. The weather is so nice.'

'You are sweet, the weather is always nice here. I would like best to stay here,' I answered markedly matter-of-factly.

'You are not serious about this, are you? I thought we'd still venture something. We could pay a spontaneous visit to Willy.'

'I didn't mean this at all. I meant, I could always remain on the island as far as the weather is concerned. However, do you really think we can suddenly appear at Willy's when we have not even told him at all that we are on the island? This is somehow embarrassing for me.'

'He'll never have any hard feelings towards us for this. He is always glad when he sees you, he almost feels like your father, and you both Dutch people understand each other really well. Moreover, he is already very old meanwhile, well over seventy, I think.'

We needed no road map of Majorca anymore. Even more we knew the way to Willy's close to Campos. Willy was a real character, a special person who had got stuck on the island many decades ago. He was actually an architect, came from Holland and spontaneously fell in love with the island. With his own hand he had built in decades of work four small summer cottages. I had got to know him in our town, because he had a friend who was resident in our quarter and spent her old age in Majorca.

He had invited us then to spend our holidays with the children in one of his bungalows. The offer was so tempting that we had then spent the whole summer holidays there and still went to him for many years. Behind Palma, leaving the highway behind the airport, we drove in our small hired car over the flat, dried out country, past old fincas with shattered water mills and old stone walls at the roadside.

This route through nature was always an optical adventure, and we always went slowly through the narrow country roads. Our common hobby is tortoises. We have three Greek ones and a Moorish tortoise at home in our garden, and here you could see some in the wild and had to pay attention that you ran over none.

We parked our car in front of the biggest house, which was also the oldest one. His old yellow Citroen stood in front of the car port under which you should best park no car anymore. It had to have been a long time since the car had been moved. The tyres were already a little flat, and the windscreens were stuck together of dust and birds' excrement. We walked around all houses. All doors were closed, the front gardens looked overgrown, and no-one could be seen.

We went over the country road to a house which Willy had rented out permanently back then. In front of it there stood an old delivery van. When we reached the house, we saw a worker at a garbage hill piling up rubble with a shovel. The face seemed familiar to us. When he saw us, he put the shovel in front of his legs and waited.

'*Buenos días, señor,* I believe I recognise you,' I said amiably. He smiled and nodded.

'We are friends of Willy's, but he is not at home,' I continued. A strange feeling came up inside of me, so that my voice was slightly trembling. He said:

'Yes, I remember you. I worked for Willy back then.'

We held our breath. We already had a bad foreboding without having spoken of what we both felt.

'Willy is dead.'

As he said it, so it was. I could not hide my wet eyes anymore and turned round and saw Willy's house.

'He already died last autumn,' he said quietly. It was not until now that I noticed he was a German, and I remembered that he had maintained the court then and would have liked best to remain on the island. He has remained. And Willy is not there anymore.

Now Beate took the floor:

'What did he die of?'

The German señor answered immediately:

'Of pancreatic cancer. He went back to Holland to have an operation. He actually wanted to remain in Holland with his children. But the doctors had given him only a few weeks more. So he came back again and still built almost half a year on his houses. His children and grandchildren were here in summer. If you want, I'll give you their address in Holland. It is lying by the phone, just as it was then.'

With Willy a part of my life had died. We sat in the car and drove the same street back to Palma. We could not talk. We drove on the highway and then past the airport.

'Tomorrow we will also be here again,' I said and desperately struggled for a normal pitch of the voice.

'The flight is only in the evening, after all,' Beate answered, somehow questioningly, 'so I will pack our bags only tomorrow morning. Today I cannot do this. Let's go by the Old Town once again later.'

'Yes, with pleasure,' I answered and felt a little easier.

## Chapter 25

Our small holiday apartment lay in the centre of Palma. It was small, but practical, had an open kitchen, and the bedroom was out to the back and quiet. When we passed through the thick walls of the entrance, the air of the Indian summer, still hot, attacked us. We lingered towards the Old Town, not because of the many restaurants, but almost no cars went there, the old Jugendstil houses cooled the heated streets and provided rest and satisfaction. Moreover, we were near the harbour, and it took only a few steps, and we could select a café in the harbour to enjoy the sundown.

We were used to going for a walk every day and talking. The mood was not as depressing anymore as in the car, but we could not get away from Willy's death.

'It is inexplicable to me. I learn about my severe kidney disease, we go to Majorca as if we were dazed and could not imagine at all that Willy could be dead. I could not grasp it at all. This totally knocks my socks off. I had concentrated so strongly on myself and my disease that I could think of nothing else anymore. I succeeded in drinking no drop of alcohol for more than one week, lived almost exclusively on fruit and salad and felt somehow better already, and now this terrible news.'

I heard how Beate took a deep breath:

'Do you still remember, three years ago when we were with Willy once? At that time he could hardly walk. He had gout in both feet and went on crutches. When we were sitting with him, he also drank nothing but this sweet mineral water. And earlier, there had been no day without wine. And at that time you have also kept up well on holiday. I am glad that now you have also realised how bad alcohol is.'

'You are right, but it is just more comfortable, and the evenings with Willy and Ilse were, after all, very romantic when the chill sea air blew over here and the crickets slowly stopped to chirp.'

'You can embellish everything by drinking. I finished with alcohol five years ago already and informed myself at that time, also because of the children. In our society things do not seem to work without alcohol. Especially youngsters are particularly endangered if in the cliques the drinking is part of the membership. Every doctor will confirm to you that alcohol is a nervous poison. I have read that up to 30,000 nerve cells die every time you are drunk.'

'Unfortunately, I must agree with you. I also once had a violent pain in the big toe, and my family doctor, who is meanwhile in retirement, asked me whether I eat a lot of grill sausages and drink beer. He told me then that the consumption of alcohol is often underestimated as a risk factor for cancer. At the same time air pollution, stress and the renunciation of fruit and vegetables is overestimated and seen as greater dangers.'

She took up this thought immediately:
'Alcohol is a drug, but hardly anyone dares to say it so clearly. Booze is simply socially acceptable. In the same vein, the possibilities of a healthy lifestyle are completely disregarded and underestimated. And what is almost always denied, alcohol is addictive. And addiction is a very bad illness. One single alcoholic in a family can destroy the whole family. For me everybody who drinks his little beer in the evening is already on the best way to become an alcoholic. And the clinics are full.'

'I do not want to contradict you at all. I know that by regular drinking of booze not only the gout risk rises, but it can also lead to inflammations of the pancreas.'

'And now we are at Willy again. To sum up, whether it sounds nice or not, but in my opinion he drunk himself to death, albeit slowly, but continuously and dead certainly. Willy could still have lived healthily for very many years. He did not smoke and moved a lot and worked outdoors on his houses. You can really be sorry for him.'

## Chapter 26

It was bright for a long time already, but was still very early. I was sitting at the kitchen table, the window was far opened, and the first living noise of the Old Town penetrated into the room. It had a reassuring effect, although I do not actually like noise. In front of me there were apples, apricots, peaches and pale green bulging grapes as you cannot paint them more nicely. And the perfume. It was intoxicating. I had never perceived such a dream of perfume. Beate was still in the bathroom, and I dwelled on my thoughts. Why was I surprised at this indescribable smell which came from the big fruit bowl? I could actually not smell right at all anymore since as a schoolboy I had worked six weeks in the colour factory. I will never forget it. At that time I was just seventeen and wanted to earn my driving licence and a small car. The hourly wage was inestimably high then. I believe at that time I had to pay no taxes as a schoolboy and could keep everything. It really had been enough for the driving licence, at that time 300 DM, and a R4 for 900 DM.

I was over the moon, but on the border to become addicted to sniffing. My job in the colour factory was on the one hand to pull colour samples from the gigantic steel barrels with a very long trowel and to clean empty barrels with some chemicals. However, the trowel did not always go down to the colour when the barrel was almost empty. I rose on a wooden footstool then and stretched over the edge of the barrel so deeply into the barrel that I was inside up to the hip. I had to breathe by force and without protective mask. I cannot remember any protective mask at all with any worker. What I inhaled had only a little in common with air. But it was not disagreeable. I got used to it fast. Since that time I liked to paint at home, the walls or the bicycle. I found the colour smell to be intoxicating. Only many years later I noticed that I could not smell so well anymore. All too often I heard:

'Don't you smell this, it stinks pathetically here!'

I smelt nothing. But this morning, this was like the resurrection of my nose. I must at once tell Beate. At that moment the door also opened.

'I can smell properly again,' I shouted to her, pleased.

'I'm pleased for you. Then just close the windows, the exhaust gas from the cars is terrible.'

'I did not mean that. The fruit, it is the fruit which smells so fantastic.'

'That always smells well. But especially here on the island. This is quite right. And you look much more recovered already, after those few days. No alcohol, this seems to agree with you fine. And in bed I saw you had struggled yourself free with the warmth so much that you have properly lost weight. You should pay attention that you eat enough, otherwise you might collapse.'

'I feel very well, however, and will destroy the fruit right now. This has to go if we are going to fly today.'

After a peach, three apricots and a big shoot with grapes I was so full that I got down nothing more. I raised and looked at my naked belly and then my legs. My small beer belly had really disappeared, and my legs, I looked at the calves, were smooth, all lacerations had healed.

I had completely forgotten about the itch of the legs. I absolutely had to report this to Beate too, but she had already disappeared in the bathroom again.

I felt well-balanced, although slowly the wistful feeling of leaving climbed up inside of me. I felt the desire to linger once again through the Old Town of Palma without any hurry. Beate still wanted to wash her hair, and this lasted just a bit longer then. I said goodbye for an hour or so and intervened disinterestedly in the diligent tumult of the inhabitants. I enjoyed the advantage not to rush after a target, to confide freely, but not drifting, in my intentions. I was not hungry, not thirsty, felt no pain, but I was not healthy, but ill, seriously ill. In a few days the appointment with the nephrologist was due. Thoughts can hardly be more bewildering, like sparks jumping to and fro between happiness and fear.

But time does not stop, and neither does thinking. I go, time goes along, my thoughts remain with me, and nevertheless everything changes, time and thinking. One hour is nothing. I have really eaten almost only fruit for one week, I could hardly believe it myself. I have drunk no alcohol for one week, no glass of fresh, bright wine, no chilled Pilsner. and that on Majorca with heavenly sunshine, blue sky and a view at the harbour and the sea.

However, was it a renunciation, a torture, a feeling of injustice because all the others drink round me and eat like crazy? Somehow not.

It was, in the first few days, unfamiliar in the literal sense, also strange, to sit in a bar and to drink water, like a leper, like one who is not part of it anymore. It was somehow difficult and depressing, but then again such a feeling of success to have made it, the first whole day on the solar island, sober. A feeling of success which carries along with it a touch of satisfaction and self-esteem. Consciousness has to do with action. The feeling of being an outsider became a feeling of the unusual.

I have become more conscious of myself in a few days. I have become attentive to myself. I have won something new by the supposed renunciation. Satisfaction. And the feeling to live more intensely. My thoughts have somehow become clearer. My brain feels lighter, brighter.

Or do I just imagine the whole thing because I see no other way out to fix my blood values again? Is it the pure fear to die suddenly of kidney failure? Do I suppress this fear by a self-deception? Does my brain play a trick on me? I have to go back, Beate is certainly waiting already.

## Chapter 27

The last day of the holidays just flew by. A ritual had developed during those many years, namely the round trip on the last day - once again heading for all important places by car, like a summary of the whole holidays, in a quick passage. This makes it easier to keep the nice time in memory, so you can somehow better conclude this period of life. We drove to Valldemosa once again, then through the winding west coast with the sharp mountain slopes on the right and the harsh cliffs on the left down to the sea till the wide plain of the north to Porto Pollensa, further to Arta and finally to Cala Figueira.

There we sat in the harbour once again with a view of the small fishing boats and drew a conclusion of our free days, and the mineral water without gas should not be missed. From there we went via Campos – Willy had lived nearby – back to Palma, to the small holiday apartment. On this way back we hardly spoke, and dwelled more on our thoughts. You must give enough time to the brain to process everything. That way only you achieve internal rest.

As we had to leave the flat in the morning, we went to bed earlier than usual, and it was good that way, because, we were very exhausted after all, by the island round trip as well as by the many impressions in this clenched form. It was still very warm and muggy. I lay down and immediately fell asleep.

'Adam,' I heard a voice over me. Did this mean me? I lifted my head, but could recognise nobody. The sky was light blue, and no cloud could be seen.

'Adam,' shouted the voice again.

'What is saddening you? You are in paradise, always remember that. And I have also created a woman for you. You should be happy.'

I looked round myself. Everything was green, birds twittered, my wife was lying beside me and sleeping, her breath was quiet, and she appeared relaxed and content. I was thinking.

'Lord, it is the apple tree of which I dreamt. Apples, so you have taught us, are the most nutritious food, they are not only healthy, but also taste as well as they look. And the nicest ones hang on a tree which we should not touch. I do not understand this, this is what my thoughts circled around in sleep.'

'This is the tree of knowledge, my son.'

'If it was the tree of misunderstanding or misfortune, or something similarly bad, I could understand it, but knowledge. This contradiction only resolves if I assume that we should not make the knowledge, that we should not know any more than we already know now. Is it really your will that we people remain silly? This I cannot imagine. I suppose something else behind it. You want to wake up our curiosity, task our brain and try out whether it works as you have created it. A brain with a creative performance which destroys customary encrustations to be able to create new things. And this is knowledge.'

'Beware of such diabolical thoughts, they will engulf you into the abyss.'

'You're putting me to the proof whether I can resist your threat and have my own will, which you created, after all, so that we are real people, with a mind and spirit. That is the solution of the problem. And the fact that you have chosen the apple and not the cherry or gooseberry, this you have answered basically yourself because in the apple there are all vital components for human beings.'

I straightened up to reach for an apple of the tree of knowledge with my right hand, when it was suddenly thundering and flashing. Soaked in sweat, I awoke, the bedroom window was open and a summer thunderstorm covered Majorca in the middle of the night.

### Chapter 28

Leaving is a little like dying, and I was always very sad when I had to leave the island. In the past, I liked to allow myself a big decanter of wine still before we went to the airport, but today? I was sober and clear in my mind, and was glad finally to be in the airplane. This time we had no window seat, that was already taken as well. After I had stowed away our hand luggage in the upper rack and had pressed shut the flap, I sat down in the middle of the triple seat, Beate took the seat at the passageway. With a friendly hello, I welcomed my neighbour, an approximately sixty-year-old man with thin, slightly grey hair, a roundish head and a slight beer belly. He was just fastening the seatbelt and was desperately searching for the latch. It was, as usual, between the seats and was too short for the waist measurement. But he seemed to know his stuff. With a few hand movements he opened the buckle and extended the belt.

'Well,' he turned his head to me and looked at my slender belly.

'Thank God you have no problems with this!'

'I will not thank God for it,' I answered. He looked at me, surprised:

'Well, it wasn't meant that way. I know myself that I must lose weight, and I won't be able to help losing weight.'

Now I looked at him questioningly. He absolutely wanted to tell me and did not even take a breath, but immediately prattled away:

'I am visiting an old friend in South America. Germany is only the stopover. My friend has invited me to a three-month trip through the Andes. There I will certainly lose weight. I cannot tell you at all how I am looking forward to it. For many years I have been waiting feverishly for this day. Now I am finally free and can do what I want.'

'Have you won the lottery or something similar?' I asked bluntly. The machine jerked, over the microphone we were asked to straighten the seats and to fasten the seatbelts. While the machine moved to the runway, the usual security instruction by a stewardess was going on. Then the machine turned, and through the round window you saw how the airplane in front of us took off. We already stood in start direction, and the engines howled, and after a few seconds our bodies were pressed to the back into the armchairs, and before you knew it, the machine already took off. The airplane lay down a little to the right and flew a big curve. Now through the window you could recognise Palma and already the next machine behind us, as it took off from the runway.

It is impressive over and over again when every two minutes an airplane starts and not rarely up to 200,000 passengers on one day are checked in. A start is always thrilling, and then in the airplane it is always totally quiet. The brighter lamps were lit again, the first newspapers rustled, small children began to cry, and the general activity took its run. The strain had subsided, and my neighbour told me his biography. He had been a medical student then, shortly before graduation, when he got the news that his uncle in Majorca had passed away and had left him his hotel. This had been 25 years ago. Now he had sold his hotel because the latest stipulations of the authorities would have ruined him.

'Haven't you regretted sometime having given up the medical studies?' I asked him.

'No, the advantages clearly predominated. It wasn't a very big hotel either, but it was directly at the beach and was very popular. We had a lot of regular customers, of course from Germany. And every time I felt the desire, I could resort to my yacht and enjoy the peace. It was quite a marvellous life.'

### Chapter 29

The flight from Majorca to Germany takes less than two hours. We had just reached the flight altitude, when the flight attendants already began to push their food box through the centre aisle. First there were the drinks. Beate and I decided on a plastic mug of mineral water, our neighbour preferred a small bottle of white wine.

With the next carriage there were, as usual, sandwiches. 'Sausage or cheese,' asked the stewardess. We three decided on cheese, and I gave my sandwich to Beate, who accepted it thankfully.

'I haven't eaten anything at all this morning,' she tried to justify herself.

'Ah, so now I know why you are so slender. If you eat nothing, you just cannot grow fat,' my neighbour grumbled, chewing and much too loud, into my ear.

'Since you are almost a medic, I can tell you that I have seriously changed my food. For one week I have been eating only fruit, for health reasons,' I answered and felt how I got excited internally.

'What do you mean, ill, you don't look like that at all.'

'Well, this can be explained in a few sentences. I was at the doctor's shortly before our one-week holiday, because of a life insurance. The lab values then showed a very strongly excessive creatinine level of the kidneys. The value was critically high, and my family doctor immediately sent me to the nephrologist, to a dialysis clinic. The appointment is in three days. I have tried to find out, in the shortness of time, as much as possible about this value and have looked for causes.

With that, it has become clear to me how important the kidneys are for the body. But I don't need to explain this to you. You also know that the main task of the kidneys is decontamination. On the other hand you can read what you want: All experts state that you cannot cure kidneys. This has quite thrown me off course. Only in one single booklet it is mentioned virtually by the way that it is possible after all, and a scientist had cured his kidneys. Namely with vitamin C in overdose. I have quite simply considered that if the kidneys are there for decontamination, they can only recover if they have nothing to do, that is they don't have to decontaminate any poisons. So I resolved to eat only food which is as free of poison as possible. And that is just fruit. And up to now I have read about no case or have heard that some-body has died of fruit!'

I trembled almost in the whole body and had got indescribably into excitement when I got everything off my chest without catching breath.

'As you say it, you are very serious about it, this can properly be felt. Admirable. I would not be able to do this. And I must admit that I also know no-one who lives only on fruit. Is this not too one-sided on a continuing basis? What about the possible deficiency symptoms then? I can imagine that other diseases will appear. Whether this is healthy on a continuing basis, I can hardly imagine.'

He really seemed to wonder.

'I don't know this yet either. But I have experi-enced visible improvements. The itch in the legs completely stopped after a few days. I sleep through the night again, and what my wife finds especially pleasant: I do not snore anymore. And I have lost several kilos, round the belly. And, I feel fit. I am cu-rious as to what the next lab values will look like.'

Deep inside I was afraid of it. But I did not say this.

'No meat? No alcohol? Nothing else?' My neighbour looked at me in disbelief.

'Right, no bread, cake, ice, pizza or noodles either. Once I tried to eat a few noodles three days ago because I became ravenously hungry, and, you can believe me or not, I had stomach cramps the whole night. This was enough for me.'

## Chapter 30

1st of October, 2010. Twice I have driven past the entrance to the parking ground of the dialysis clinic and turned round over and over again after some metres. Either I was so much in fear and thought, or my inside controlled me so much that, subconsciously controlled, I simply did not want to drive there. After the parking I took the lift.

There it was written in black thick letters: Dialysis – reception. I entered and stood in front of a big, almost chest-high bar, and nobody welcomed me. The ladies in white behind the bar not even looked up, they were making phone calls or stared into the computer like petrified. By request I mentioned my name and all important things which you had to reveal at such a registration, and then I was sent to the waiting room. After a few minutes I was picked up by an assistant and was led into a very narrow room. My size was registered at 176 cm and was taken down, and then I had to go on the scales: 69 kilos. I could see it myself between my feet. Nine kilos less than two weeks ago, shortly before our Majorca holiday. So little I had weighed at the age of 20 years. Then several amounts of blood were also taken from me. And I did not faint.

As a student I often donated blood. This brought 50 DM every time and an opulent meal in the university clinic. At that time this was a lot of money. My student digs cost only 120 DM per month. With the blood donation I had got used to look as the needle was pricked into the skin. It is quite strange what you get used to, even if it hurts a little. According to the assistant's opinion, even strong men have supposedly fainted. Then of course you feel super-duper and leave the doctor's office, your chest swollen with pride.

Then I had to wait again. I had got over the first hurdle, now there was yet the conversation with the doctor, the boss and specialist, the so-called nephrologist. Now I noticed that I sweated very much after all, although a fresh breeze flowed out by the tilting window and the autumn air was pleasantly chilly. I felt hot. Another assistant came and got me.

'Please come this way, the last door on the right.'

The hallway was white and long. I knocked, heard a voice and entered.

There he sat, the specialist, white coat, white shirt, tie, small head with a high forehead, a short man behind a huge desk which was almost empty.

'Please have a seat,' he certainly must have said. I cannot remember anymore. Anyway, I sat in front of him and he looked at a printed sheet of paper. He got the lab results from my doctor, he said, and that this was very serious indeed. But they wanted to order a comprehensive new laboratory examination, and therefore they had taken several vials of blood from me. Before I left the office, I should still take a big bottle for collecting urine, and I would also get a blood pressure monitor installed, which stores the blood pressure for 24 hours. So far I was able to endure everything well, and then I had to give an account of my profession.

From financial need I had had to change my sources of income over and over again, had learnt a total of three occupations with final examinations and had worked my way up over and over again:

This had strengthened my self-confidence rather than unnerved me. I always had stress, without a question, and it had not become less during the last few years either.

Dr Duesberg pulled an empty A4 paper from the drawer, put it down crosswise in front of himself, twisted a pencil from his white breast pocket like a magician and slowly drew a long line straight across the paper, almost like a diagonal from the left below to the right on top, and he murmured:

'I suppose you have a chronic renal insufficiency, which, as the line shows here on the paper, slowly rises higher and higher and then sometime, all of a sudden...', the pencil abruptly went vertically down almost to the edge of the sheet and left a terrible deep abyss,

'… there's the end.'

I must have visibly winced. He immediately went on speaking:

'You appear very healthy otherwise. You are an ideal candidate for a kidney transplant.'

All perceptible muscles of my body cramped into concrete. I had thought about dialysis, had dreamt of it, had rejected quite a lot of thoughts of it again or had suppressed them, but a transplant, no, I had not thought of that at all.

Why, actually? Why had I not come across this thought myself? I had read or heard that hundreds of patients are waiting for a donator's kidney for many years. So maybe that is why I completely cut out this measure from my considerations. I do not know anymore what my thoughts were, all at once. But I still know exactly what I answered to him when I had overcome the state of shock:

'I have completely changed my food. For nearly two weeks I have been eating only fruit, bio-fruit.'

My voice trembled. I did not know myself at all that way.

'Such a diet is not disadvantageous, but it is no healing. You cannot always pull yourself up by your own bootstraps.'

This was too much of everything. I really began to doubt myself. However, at the same time I also felt an internal resistance.

'Doctor, what I do is no diet, it is a basic food change!'

I had the impression to have spoken especially loudly, but it was very quiet. Nevertheless, he must have heard it, because he recapitulated as regards contents:

'With a diet you cannot heal your advanced renal insufficiency.'

He got up and gave me his small hand. I had certainly left the consulting room shakily. The assistants gave me the uric bottle, the blood pressure measuring instrument and a new appointment to take with me on my way home, and a small stub of paper with the new discussion appointment in three days.

### Chapter 31

Beate sat in the kitchen on her usual place and looked by the terrace door in the garden.

'Well? What did he say?'

I sat down opposite her and told in a quiet tone what the specialist, a nephrologist by his trade, had said. I must have appeared very low-spirited, because she started to comfort me:

'We have gone through a lot already, we will still make this. You will go again soon, maybe the values are not so bad at all, and now you're beating yourself up more than necessary. Rest for the moment. The transplant will not happen all that fast. And should it really come this far, I'll also have my kidneys checked as to what is possible.'

'I know you would do everything for me, but I must first of all digest all that now. And that he always only speaks of a diet, as if he had not listened properly. I said it clearly enough, though, and also repeated it. I simply do not understand this, when it is proved that nutrition is so important, if not even vital.'

To which she said:

'Many doctors have no or little knowledge about nutrition. Maybe you should also visit a medical practicioner once. I have gained some good experience there earlier with the children.'

'I don't know, this is too unscientific for me and is afflicted too much with the problem of placebo. I trust these people still less. I am not religious enough for it.'

I slowly walked into my room and lay down on the sofa. I was so exhausted that I soon fell asleep. When I woke, it was already getting dark. I had to go to the toilet, and when I entered the small bright room, I saw the big yellowish plastic bottle. Every time, the whole night and the next day till the evening the bottle filled, almost up to the lid. It felt warm, and I was surprised how much urine you deliver in such a short time. Somehow I had the feeling I had something of me in my hand. On the right upper arm I had attached the blood pressure measuring instrument. At irregular intervals it blew up hard and slowly pulled itself together again. At night I had woken several times because of it, and I even had only slept lying on one side. Each time I wanted to turn round mechanically, the device prevented me from doing so. Then I had woken up and had remained lying on the back to fall asleep again. The next morning I felt as if broken on the wheel. Late in the afternoon I brought the uric bottle and the measuring instrument back to the dialysis clinic. The next appointment was in two days. I simply did not want to remember and took Wandmaker's book up again. I had meanwhile arrived on page 130:

'Doctors get paid nothing for health **information**. No wonder they are gradually fed up with this instruction not at all desired from their patients. We can, however,  put one thing into action immediately: namely at least supply a lot of vitamin C as the most important vitamin supplement! Vitamins are healthy and have hardly any side effects even in high doses – in contrast to many harmful prescription drugs. For decades, his colleagues insinuated that with the vitamin C, *Pauling* only produced kidney stones and expensive urine. The American biochemist was able to produce the evidence towards his critics that 85 percent of the additional vitamin C remain in the body and only 15 percent are eliminated by way of the urine. Thus the organism always disposes of an extensive vitamin C depot, and no kidney stones will be formed either. On the contrary

– the function of the kidneys improves considerably after the supply of vitamin C. *Pauling* further found out that after a regular intake of large amounts of vitamin C, he had to suffer neither from colds nor from indigestion.

Vitamin C is, besides, the cheapest and most acceptable lubricant for our bowels. You get an obstipation only from a diet of dead animals and viscous grains. The usual laxatives lead to addiction and to considerable losses of electrolytes as well as of the most important mineral substances potassium and magnesium, which are antagonists of the calcium. *Pauling* put the weight of the dog in relation to that of one person and determined that we would have to take in **360 oranges containing vitamin C** daily to be able to catch up with the dog's ability to form vitamin C by itself. So he first began with four to five grams of vitamin C powder and increased the dosis to **18 grams** at last, **which means 18,000 milligrams every day**!! *Pauling* calls vitamin C the protective vitamin against all heart and circulatory discomfort and even against cancer. That way he was able to keep his prostate cancer, latent for 30 years already, in check up to his 93$^{rd}$ year – he passed away in 1994.'

My effervescent tablets with vitamin C from Majorca were used up. I put the book aside and directly went to the next chemist's shop in our quarter.

I asked for vitamin C and was again showed these plastic tubes with the vitamin tablets in different flavours.

'I have read that there is very inexpensive vitamin C!' 'Yes, wait a moment,' said the young shop assistant with a granny's knot in the back of her head and disappeared behind the antique sliding door. When she appeared again, she laid a small round little jar out to me on the bar with the remark: 'You may not take too much of it, however. That will be two euros and 70.' I thanked, and she must have seen that I shook my head. On one hand I had read something completely different shortly before, on the other hand the price was negligibly low in proportion to the effervescent tablets. You should not take too much of it? Is she just so silly and uneducated or was she really serious about such a nonsense and maybe has even learnt it in her education? I could not imagine that Wandmaker should have made up his evidence.

### Chapter 32

It was more and more difficult for me to live only on fruit. I did not seem to need vast amounts of energy, because every spare minute I sat in front of the PC and kept on trying to find out as much as possible about the kidneys and their job in the body. When I stared intensely into the flat panel display, I noticed neither the strain nor the tiredness, but I heard my stomach growling more and more. I felt visibly weaker, and regularly and more and more often I lay down on the bed.

The shock which Dr Duesberg had administered to me was effective. I became more and more scared. Should he really be right, I was closer to death than to life. At the same time I resisted internally to give up my conviction to relieve my kidneys with the radical food change to fruit and vegetables and to offer them the freedom to recover. And if I am absolutely wrong and it gets worse and worse?

I do not want to die, and I do not want to go to the dialysis. I became more and more insecure what I was more afraid of, that the doctor was right and my food change was only a self-deception, or did I have a bigger fear of the dialysis, so that I was wandering on a wrong path which led me to the downfall? What should I really stick to, what could I conform to?

Today I had asked my wife to cook jacket potatoes, without salt, to be sure, and corn salad with lemon and a little cold-pressed olive oil from the wholefood shop. I had well tucked in, I had not eaten such a serving for two weeks anymore. It was pleasing for me that I had taken pleasure in the taste of the potatoes. They tasted somehow properly of potatoes and not of salt. However, after lunch I had to lie down again. My body felt a strange load, and I believed to feel how the blood flowed out of the fingers into the stomach. My after-lunch sleep was short, but full of nightmares.

I lay on the back and stared at the wall. I began to speak to myself with an internal voice: You are on the right track. You have achieved something that nobody would have expected of you: Two weeks of no meat, no bread, no cheese, no coffee, no tea and no drop of alcohol. Fear is and remains the strongest driving force with a human being. I knew this. The prospect to get something good is not as immense by a long shot as the fear to lose something. I tried to concentrate again. What else have I done differently during the last two weeks ? I have massively diminished my professional stress. But I will not be able to keep this up further.

Meanwhile I felt the panic grow in me, because our reserve was already used up, and I was forced to acquire new customers again. The stress will go on, whether I want it or not. What else has happened? I thought intensely. Then it occurred to me when I stretched a leg to the ceiling: The itch had stopped. And how I had still scratched my calves bloody a few weeks ago. Now nothing at all anymore, the wounds had even already healed. This must be a huge progress, though. This cannot just be by chance. I did not imagine this. And my knees! Already on Majorca it had struck my wife that I did not lament about knee pain anymore. My knees were quite simply painless.

Or did I want to imagine this too? Thinking had upset me so strongly again that I had almost fallen asleep again. Half asleep, I observed my legs in my mind's eye. They would actually have to start to tremble now. But nothing happened. For many years already, my legs always started to tremble, shortly before falling asleep, as if one inflicted small electric shocks to them. I had traced this back to my stress. But now I felt relaxation in my legs.

Something has happened in my body. This had not necessarily to have to do with the kidneys, and maybe the alcohol was the cause. Booze is a nervous poison, that is just how it is. I was really glad not to feel my legs. I woke up and drew a little confidence again. Tomorrow I will have to go to Dr Duesberg again. The fear, it crawled up in me again.

## Chapter 33

When I woke, the alarm clock was ringing. It took some seconds until I was so awake that I could get up and turned off the alarm clock. It was still early. Beate had also woken and looked at me, surprised.

'I could not sleep half of the night. You will go to the doctor again shortly. I did not want to wake you. You were asleep so soundly that I asked myself: How can he be so fast asleep when he has to go to the doctor again tomorrow? You certainly will be informed of your new values. I believe you have slept through the whole night.'

I pondered:

'Yes, I also believe I did not once go to the toilet. This is the first time since... I do not know at all how long it is that I did not have to get up the whole night. Actually, when I think about the days and nights, I must realise that it became less and less that I had to go out at night. This can only be due to the food change. To what else? Patients with kidney diseases have to go out at night often, this I have read. I had decided, though, to drink even more water at night too. But if you sleep, this is not possible, of course.'

While she also rose, she said casually:

'You should discuss this with the doctor sometime. But I also think that this is a progress.'

The appointment was at 10 o'clock. I was immediately called in and sat quite tensely in front of the big, almost empty desk with the short doctor behind it.

'Your lab values have come. Since I know that you want to check and read everything yourself, I have made a copy for you. Then you can take them with you. Have a look.'

With his left hand he slipped the copy to me over the table, and with his right hand, extended by his pencil, he pointed at a number in boldface type with an exclamation mark behind it. I put on my reading glasses and quietly read the number:

'Four point one, one.'

'This is your creatinine level. It would be normal around one. More than four is the last, the fourth stage. Also other blood values have immensely got out of hand.'

He paused his breathing, as if he did not want to breathe anymore, and looked directly into my eyes. I slowly dropped my eyes, not so much in order to avoid him, but rather in order to think. I must probably have looked like a picture of misery. In any case, I was tongue-tied. However, I wanted to tell him that I slept the whole night through, maybe even the first time for many years. I said nothing.

'Your diet will not help you there anymore. I already told you this.' His tone appeared more harsh. I wanted to answer that it is not question of a diet, but a food change. But I was quiet. The doctor interrupted the silence:

'In one week at the same time we will meet again here.' I looked up to him, directly into his clear, bright eyes.

'Till then you will have decided, so in exactly one week, whether you stick to your diet or, as I have already told you as well, take up dialysis.'

He rose jerkily and stretched his right hand out to me straight across the big desk. I got up as well, pressed his little hand, took the slip of paper with the lab values.

'Here is also a copy of the letter to your family doctor, give him my regards, the original will be sent to him,' he added.

I took everything and wanted to leave the room, however turned round once again and asked:

'May I, actually, do sport?'

'Certainly,' he returned, 'but you should not exaggerate.'

## Chapter 34

'You are all white in your face, and you have bags under your eyes.' This is how I was received, although I had not properly entered the hall at all.

'Is it so bad?' she asked directly afterwards.

'Let's go to the kitchen, I must first of all drink a glass of water.'

I sat down to the massive wooden table and spread out the pages in front of myself.

'The covering letter encloses two pages in small print, and the lab values also fit exactly on two pages. I'll just count over something.'

I took a ballpoint pen and tapped successively on all values which were outside the norm and were furnished with an exclamation mark.

23 values are down the drain. I shook my head and could pronounce the sentence only in fragments.

'Here, just you read the letter.'

She took both pages.

'Read out to me everything loudly and slowly. I want to understand everything, no matter how cruel it is.'

And she began to read:

'Dear colleague – this certainly means Dr von Rothenburg. Now a lot of abbreviations follow, such as SYST: 162 mmHg and so on. Here,'

she flipped the following side open:

'It is written here: Diagnosis: now it comes: Iron deficiency anaemia, renal anaemia, secondary hyperparathyreoidism, arterial hypertension and chronic renal insufficiency, stage four. Below here further below: Evaluation and proposal of treatment. On account of the proteinuria it is to be assumed a chronically progressive glomerular damage of unclear genesis with preexisting chronic renal insufficiency.' She read on in a whisper, probably to leave out the foreign words which will not help us a lot right away, and continued loudly:

'because of the iron deficiency anaemia, moreover, a short-term check whether a slow progression is continuously present or is accelerating. In the end there is something written of a renal biopsy.'

She breathed deeply. We looked at each other and were quiet. I would preferably have burst out crying. I stood up and wanted to go to my room. I wanted to be for myself. Completely alone. I turned once more to her and stammered:

'I must have decided till next week. Then I'll have to go to the dialysis immediately, the doctor believes. My fruit has failed. I don't want this anymore. I can't bear this anymore.'

I walked into my room and lay down on the couch. I was exhausted like never before in my life. I had a thick head, and in my ears the tinnintus squeaked for its life. I must probably have fallen asleep somehow. When I opened my eyes, it was already almost dark, and Beate was standing in front of me.

'You can live with dialysis. And it can also help. This doesn't have to be for good. We'll make this all right.'

'You mean well, but I can't come to terms with it. I simply don't want this, do you understand? I don't want it. I hate dependence. I won't stand this.' I was excited and already shouted so loud that she tried to calm me.

'Maybe you should seek another opinion after all, I mean from another doctor. Just ask our family doctor whether he knows yet other specialists.'

Although with this proposal nothing changed in the state of affairs, I felt the first signs of smallest possible hope.

'Yes. Now it is already too late. I'll call immediately tomorrow morning . Of course. I will do this in any case. Quite clearly.'

### Chapter 35

'Dr Grevenbeck and his colleague, his name just doesn't occur to me, this would still be a very good address. For many years they've had a very much approved dialysis clinic.'

On the phone the voice of my family doctor sounded unexpectedly friendly and positive, as if he was not surprised at all that I asked for another recommendation, although the first recommendation also came from him. In any case, I thanked in a friendly way and immediately, without hesitating, dialled the phone number passed on to me.

'The next free appointment with Dr Grevenbeck is the 15th of October, immediately in the morning around eight,' answered a thin, squeaky ladies' voice. I agreed to the appointment, of course, and was even glad, which, however, surprised me in turn, because I really had no reason to be glad. Human beings live and think in relations. This had been a commonplace for me for a long time. But in this case I even had to smile about myself.

'Thus also with small things one can
Give pleasure to officials' children,'

that was an old saying from my childhood. My father was an official, which was not my fault, however.

It was still very early in the day, too early to call customers. I went online again to work on my professional emails.

From the beginning I was a customer at T-Online. To get into my email accounts, I always went by the title page. It had struck me several times already that T-Online maintained a frame with medical news and took up another medical subject in short form every few days.

'I am curious as to when they will have some news about renal insufficiency,' I said to myself and wrote the word into the empty bar of the search engine: renal insufficiency.

Besides many similar terms there was written: The therapy of renal insufficiency. I clicked on the place full of expectations and came onto the page: www.curado.de. I read:

'In most cases, however, the cause of a chronic renal insufficiency cannot be repaired, because many of the basic illnesses are not remediable. However, a good blood glucose setting with diabetics already helps, for example, to put off or to prevent a decline of the kidney function. With hypotonic people, the normalisation of the blood pressure is important. In the final stage of a chronic renal insufficiency, however, the artificial cleaning of the blood by dialysis is mostly unavoidable.'

I leant back and started to think. Text analysis was rather the specialty of my wife. The last sentence would have properly knocked my socks off if there had not been written before:
... to put off or to prevent a decline of the kidney function...
From this statement I concluded easily and unequivocally that the kidneys 'move', that something can be done at all. Up to now I had desperately looked for information about whether sick kidneys are basically remediable. I had found nothing, absolutely nothing, on the internet. Now here a first very small hint. The view suggested itself to me that in medicine, the investigation of kidney healing is not even taken into consideration at all. As a radical solution, it is always only written dialysis or transplant. As I have got to know somewhere and sometime, a

dialysis should cost about 30,000 € a year per patient.

This is a lot, a lot of money. I do not want to forecast at all what profit a dialysis clinic achieves with maybe 20 to 30 patients, whose invoices are paid without delay by the health insurance funds. With this, I am not surprised that more and more dialysis clinics come into existence. As a dialysis patient, you are not bound to your home town anymore, you can also go on holiday in Majorca and make use of the dialysis there.

'No more reading and television – fit with dialysis!' yet another article at www.curado.de.


I skimmed over this article literally on the fly. There it is reported that in one dialysis clinic the patients are offered sport during the dialysis of several hours. Even 70-year-old retirees become fit again and gain in joy of life.

'Sport means quality of life' is one of the headings, and it is written further:

'Persons suffering from chronic kidney disease who regularly do sports or maybe kinesitherapeutic exercises or moderate strength training profit in many respects: medically, socially and economically.'

Unfortunately, the medical effects were not further explained. When I read this, I remembered that Dr Duesberg had not advised against sport. I used to play indoor football and volleyball with pleasure, and was even enrolled in a fitness studio for a while. In the afternoon I read out the text passages from the internet to my wife. I had printed out the pages and had filed them away in a folder.

'By the way, our son has not taken his dumbbells with him when he moved to Düsseldorf. I have still seen them a few days ago when I cleaned the dust in his room.'

I didn't need to be told twice. I did not have to look for a long time either. There were two 5-kilo-dumbbells. They lay under the bed.

## Chapter 36

After the early morning shower I stood in underwear in my room, and the dumbbells lay in front of my feet. I raised them slowly. And stemmed them along the head to the ceiling. I repeated this several times and felt how heavy 5 kilos can suddenly become. I had only a few exercises from the fitness training in memory. I did not feel a lot of joy with my exercises. I wanted to get professional advice. In the course of the morning I went online again and looked for dumbbell exercises. However, I came across something else:

'Www.symptome.ch'

– that is the page of the forum. I do not remember at all how I came across this page. But if you surf the internet with fear and desperation and look for solutions which are apparently not there, you click on everything which gives only a hint of a solution.

Www.symtome.ch from Switzerland. Well, at least they write in German. I log in. After some confusion I had made it, now I could join the discussion. I am in a chat. This was actually something to me in which pubescent girls hang out and torment the keys, at which the German language is ruined very much, however they understand what others write, I think, because our daughter is always with it. The anonymity is there, and nevertheless somehow dissolved. I write quite simply so that everybody can just understand.

I state my size, my weight, that I was at the doctor's, who had sent me to the specialist. For the first time I wrote the word creatinine and the findings: 4.1, the fourth and last stage of a chronic renal insufficiency. While I wrote it, I felt distance, distance to myself. It was someone else who pressed the keys, not me. I was totally quiet. The writer wrote and thought only of writing everything properly, of not misspelling any words, of making no grammar mistakes in any case – they should not believe I was not educated. I wanted to find out something, but not present myself as silly.

Vanity – shortly before death. In the brain, all feelings collide, and the fingertips fall on the keys as if by themselves. This is not me, though – yes, I am me. I write about myself, somehow away from me. I am mortally ill and write to people whom I have never seen and do not know at all, and I write about my illness. But only a few sentences come out of it.

I read through them once again and had to realise it was very little and quite scarce, and something lacked. I still had sort of hope, though, which, as is generally known, dies last. I had changed my food and had started eating quite a lot of fruit. I wrote this in the end. Well. Now send off.

OK. And wait. It was quite late in the evening. So few sentences, and I felt worn out. The next morning, no coffee, no bread, three freshly squeezed oranges from the wholefood market, I switched on my PC as usual to retrieve my emails. What was this? An email from Symptome.ch. My heart was pounding up to my neck. Why was I so excited all of a sudden? I felt silly, but could not suppress my excitement and went on Enter.

There was the first message:

'Hello, Dieter'.

I had used no pseudonym. Typical. But I had not given my surname. Many are called Dieter, if not to say that it is a commonplace name. 'Hello, Dieter, your information yields a BMI of 22.6. Unfortunately, you have pursued your food change at the expense of your muscles. Fruit and nuts are poison with your kidney values (potassium and phosphate). You still have a kidney function of approx. 17%. The result is massive restrictions of the decontamination performance and a lack of resorption of important materials via the kidney, and a lot more.

A renal insufficiency goes along with a destruction of the fine nephritic filters and, hence, is not reversible. Trust your nephrologist and find out about the possibilities of the kidney replacement therapy. Shutting your eyes will be of no use, it only aggravates your situation with considerable secondary damages. For your info: www.dialyse-online.de. It is important, also in your situation, to take in enough egg white (approx. 0.7 g / kg of KG), and of course also enough energy in the form of fat and carbohydrates. Peter'

## Chapter 37

At this point, so I can imagine, there would certainly be many people who stop now, maybe even break down and surrender. It is still ringing in my ears:

'You cannot always pull yourself up by your own bootstraps.'

This was my nephrologist. To him I should go back and surrender, trust him blindly. Should I stop thinking, fighting? This is not and never was my nature. But there grew doubts in me, as tremendous as sequoias. Kidney replacement therapy. A long, apparently harmless word for a slow death. No. Or yes. Is it really the one chance? There are plenty of acquaintances who are 'stuck' to the dialysis. And they are alive. In my mind's eye I prepared to go to the dialysis clinic three times a week or more often.

I saw myself lying in bed, for hours, connected with tubes, without moving, 'chained' like a slave. I felt sick in my stomach. My throat became dry. I switched off the computer. I was knocked out. I lay down on the couch and pulled the snug cover over my shoulders and over my head. I felt what I had not felt for a long time anymore, tears. My hands were cold. My feet were cold. On my back the skin contracted. My backbone somehow trembled inwards. I tried to breathe deeper and more slowly. I looked for clear thoughts. First of all come to rest.

Rest? I was excited, wide awake and completely exhausted at the same time. Pictures from my childhood came up, small fragments of films.

I smell the fresh, juicy grass, which is higher than me. I lie on my back and look relaxedly into the blue sky. The snow-white little clouds are floating very slowly, and right in the middle my kite with its wide blue shoulders. The lower triangle was red. Red kite paper, almost transparent. Blue and red one was, at that time, only available in Holland, in the tool shop in which my grandpa stocked up with hammer and pliers for his work. And there were fishing rods there and mason's lacing cord. It did not break. My kites were gigantic, as big as me, and the span like my outstretched arms. The wind was steady in Holland, not far from the North Sea. My kite stood, the heavy tape sagged hundreds of metres, until it abruptly moved upwards. I had bound it to a thick wooden post. I lay on my back and looked relaxedly to the kite.

It stood quietly. I sniffed the smell of cows, crickets shouted for their lives, and now and again this mooing. The high grass moved like waves on a lake. Light gusts of wind stroked the grass tips.

I felt the wind on my face. It was warm, but not hot, pleasant. Every year during the summer holidays I was with granny and grandpa in Holland, in the countryside, for six weeks, the whole holidays, free.

Only granny, grandpa and I. I stopped freezing. My breath became quieter. I had cried.

**Chapter 38**

I do not remember how I spent the evening, mostly in front of the television, news, some quiz show, news of the day, but no beer, no wine. Water. The next morning, I had to answer my customer emails, and if there were any enquiries for an appointment, I wanted to call them off. I had no strength to talk to anybody in such a state, to listen to their superficial luxury problems, to surround myself with people who circle only round themselves. More than twenty new mails, and many were only advertising. I began my usual deleting practise.

There! Symptome.ch.

'You have a new email. Click here.'

I pushed the cursor on it:

"Hello, Kayen, besides, this forum is called: The end of the symptom fight. Warm greetings, Peter.'

So they had already talked about me, look there. So Kayen was also one from the chat, and now I recognise that he only cited Peter with the sentence. I am excited. I read on:

'I find this tip virtually stupid now, and you could really have refrained from it.

A food change has nothing to do with a symptom fight and is absolutely able to cure some illnesses.

Hello, Dieter, I wish for you that you can do something with the food tips already received, and that maybe you will receive many more tips helping you. Best regards, Kayen.'

### Chapter 39

One day later. I am sitting in front of the computer again and open my mailbox. Symptome.ch - a new mail! Click.

Peter writes:

'Dear Dieter, I quite understand that you have hopes not to get to the kidney replacement therapy. However, I think it is better to accept this illness and to live with it. According to Nietzsche, 'The Big Health'. The report cited by you refers to the acute renal insufficiency. You have a chronic renal insufficiency; unfortunately, these statements are not valid for it. ACE inhibitors reduce the blood pressure and can possibly delay the renal insufficiency, so can vitamin D. There is an acute renal insufficiency after burns, big surgeries, sometimes also after pregnancies or a sepsis.

Your food is rich in alkalis, hence you have no acidaemia, but, due to the missing protein, a protein energy lack, which precisely in predialysis means a raised risk of mortality. See. Http://sundoc.bibliothek.uni-halle.de... Page 3 Malnutrion.'

Peter.

Should it have been this? Peter seems to know a lot very well about the problem. What he writes is the opposite of reassuring. So what I do is a risk of mortality. Is this supposed to mean that I endanger myself even more, even risk my life if I increasingly eat fruit?

Does he want to frighten me even more? Up to now, I have not read anything about acidification. And then his hint at science!

Does it become more right this way? For me there is no free and independent science. But he seems to be in earnest. I feel strongly affected after all. Nevertheless, resistance arises in me somehow. Or do I just not want to admit it to myself? I feel helpless.

I do not want to surrender. I will not surrender. I dig deeper and continue to search – on the internet.

## Chapter 40

And I had found something. Hope mingled in my excitement. I wrote it into the net immediately:

'Honoured friends: Here, for example, I have found something:

There are doctors who deal with the regeneration of kidneys. It is interesting, among other things, that there are hardly attempts to influence nephritic damages, also chronic ones, positively. Here is the quotation:

'The scholarship holder Dr Florian Grahammer, active in the institute of internal medicine IV nephrology and general medicine at the university clinic of Freiburg, investigates mechanisms for the restoration of the function of the diseased kidney. In almost all kidney diseases, specialised cells of the nephritic filter, so-called podocytes, are concerned.

While the causes which lead to the kidney failure are partially explained, hardly anything is known to this day about the molecular processes of the restoration of the filter function of the kidney. This is also reflected in the almost complete absence of specific therapies for the treatment of kidney diseases. Preliminary works of Dr Florian Grahammer point to the fact that specialised cell-cell contacts play a crucial role also for the regeneration of the nephritic filter.

The planned molecular and cytological analysis of the function and change of these cell-cell contacts during the damage and regeneration of the nephritic filter allows to expect absolutely new insights, which could lay the foundation for restoring attempts of treatment! – this is what the Else Kröner-Fresenius foundation for the evaluation of scientific work says.'

Dieter

## Chapter 41

This had to be a nasty shock for Peter. Internally I was even a little pleased. I do not know whether Peter from the Symptome chat is a doctor or something similar. Definitely, he is very well-read, in any case he likes to chat and he also always answers immediately.

Does he maybe have to do nothing else? Maybe he sits in a wheel chair and has much more illnesses and worries than me and therefore knows a lot so well. But somehow his comments come across as a little aggressive to me, even devastating if I let them sink in at rest. Does he want to prove anything to himself and me? I am curious as to what will come now in the chat.

For the first time I have discovered information which is absolutely contrary to all opinions and statements. Finally, experts argue about the problem of a kidney healing. This gives hope. If you, dear readers, have followed me up to this point, maybe you have even looked on the Internet yourselves and have visited Symptome.ch. Nothing is extinguished there if it is not quite violating human dignity and unobjective or is abused for self-advertising. Hence, you are able to read up my chat correspondence independently.

After I have stumbled across this research approach, I gained hope, although I exactly knew that such research would take years, if not decades, until some methods are really applied to the patient.

But it was a first **Yes**.

Yes to healing, the first turning away from the irrefutable – almost God-given incurability and dialysis, a turn to ending the helplessness – and suddenly you do not feel all alone anymore. Only me alone against the whole world of dialysis doctors. I must be taken for mad, for arrogant and haughty.

One must think the impossible and do the possible, thus or similarly it was once formulated by Hermann Hesse.

But maybe I also was afraid of being laughed at and not to be taken seriously, and therefore have spoken about it with no other person, except with my wife.

Now for one week I have the diagnosis that my kidney values are life-menacingly 'down the drain', and up to now there was no reasonable approach of an effective therapy. There was only the hint from and via Helmut Wandmaker that essentially only fruit and vegetables should promote our healing and one should escape from all poisons.

This was still very vague for me up to this point and comparable rather to a straw to which I held on for the time being.

## Chapter 42

In the meantime I had become very courageous and had called off the appointment with the pistol to my head with Dr Drügeberg. On the 15th of October I will have the first appointment with Dr Grevenbeck. I am already curious a little as to how this nephrologist will react to my food change. But till then there are still a few more days.

I had decided to go in for more sports. I used to jog sometimes already, and it did not hurt. My own humour is quite strange, but I had the feeling just to resume it simply.

Right down in the cupboard I still found old sports trousers and T-shirts. I sometimes wore my sneakers for walking. They were not the most modern ones anymore either. Today I did not take a shower in the morning, but put on my old sports set, drank a glass of natural mineral water and went to my car. I was glad that no neighbours saw me. My appearance seemed quite strange enough to myself.

So I went to the canal and parked at the first bridge. I wanted to jog up to the next one. Notabene, I wanted, but already after two minutes I felt stings in the back, and my heart was in my mouth, and I began to sweat extremely. The remaining ca. 500 metres I only walked. At the next bridge I turned back and sat down on a bench and looked behind the cargo ships. Then I tried once more to begin my way back at a faster pace, which probably lasted no longer than one minute either, and I slowly trotted back to the car.

I had forced myself to try it, I could be proud of it, the rest was a fiasco. But it also led to a crystal-clear realisation: I was absolutely unfit. Self-awareness is generally said to be the first step towards improvement.

After showering I squeezed, like every morning for two weeks, several oranges. Then I took the vitamin C jar from the cupboard and, with the small transparent plastic spoon, tilted two units into the glass. Every spoon included exactly 1 gram.

After the office work and a lunch with potatoes, fresh paprika and curd I lay down on the couch again for the after-lunch sleep. I simply took the liberty of sleeping at least half an hour every noon. If I did not do it, I could not concentrate the whole afternoon and felt tired very fast again.

This afternoon my wife wanted to do some shopping in town, and I accompanied her. In the bookshop I had fast found something: A book with representations of the dumbbell training. Come home, I took two recovered dumbbells of our son's and tried some exercises.

Doing this, I developed the following order:

I took both dumbbells in my hands and hung them very deeply in front of my feet. Then I raised them slowly, so that I felt the strain in the back. With this, I raised the dumbbells only up to the upper thighs to lower them again slowly then. This practise is good for the back muscles. Then I stood up straight, the legs in a normal step position, and pulled the dumbbells on the left and on the right of me until they were under the shoulders. This I did only twice as well because here muscles are moved which you do not need so often. Then the dumbbells hung down again, and I raised them slowly in front of myself without moving the upper arms, until the forearms were in parallel with the ground, not higher, and slowly lowered them again. Then I laid the dumbbells onto my shoulders left and right and held on to them.

With that, I slowly went to my knees as deeply as I was capable of, and stretched me back into the standing position again. Now I felt my thighs immensely, though. As the last exercise I pressed, still standing, the dumbbells from the shoulder upwards to the ceiling and left them again so deeply down that the upper arms were in parallel with ground. From this tense position I pressed the dumbbells to the ceiling again.

I succeeded to do this twice, and I was exhausted. While I undertook these attempts, I developed the idea how I could measure a possible increase in performance. I decided to carry out this sequence every morning and every evening, and to raise the number of repetitions slowly.

The next morning it was time again: First a glass of natural mineral water, briefly to the toilet, then three oranges squeezed and two grams of vitamin C, and off to my room where the dumbbells were already prepared.

I had decided to repeat every single exercise three times. Every third time was pure torture, particularly the stretching from the squat with the dumbbells on the shoulder.

My legs had already become very thin, by the many years' work at the desk.

I had forgotten about the jogging for the time being. It took too much time from me and was too complicated for me. The more energy I put into the dumbbell training. After three days I already made five stages with every exercise. Then after the exercises I went to the kitchen, always highly content, to sit down with Beate, who enjoyed her breakfast coffee. Every morning I could proudly report an increase to her. On the 14th of October I had cracked the mark of ten repetitions.

On the 15th of October I cancelled the training and went, internally agitated, to the dialysis clinic of Dr Grevenbeck.

**Chapter 43**

On the way to the second dialysis clinic – I was sitting in the car – I still remembered the conversation with Beate the evening before. Obedience to authority was such a subject which had very strongly preoccupied us. Especially I had braced myself against authorities all my life.

We people obey authorities without sense and morality. My father was a police officer, and I went to a school which was led by Catholic missionaries. Very early on I recognised that you should question authorities.

Many too many people assume without a check that these people know more and can do more than we do. I had firmly decided not to let myself impress any more in such a way as last time. I wanted to ask more questions and represent my position better.

Dr Grevenbeck was much younger than I had supposed, and remarkably friendly. He thought it would make sense to have another lab check done. He reckoned we would not need all values anymore, and he looked at the lab values which I had handed over to him. I asked him about the risks with the dialysis, and what I found out here encouraged me in my steadfast wish not to have to be connected to the dialysis.

There would be a wide range of risks, he explained to me, and I must confess that I could not remember everything anymore. But one representation had remained in my brain very vividly: At the edges of likelihoods there can be very big problems, and the chances of survival are not so rosy by a long shot as it is liked to be seen in public.

To me it became clear that dialysis is not an unlimited life alternative, but always holds the mortal danger in itself. Actually, so he explained, among other things, a dialysis patient would have to hang on to the dialysis 24 hours per day. But then they would have no more quality of life, so that one would have settled for three times per week. And then came the moment when I started reporting about my food change. He listened to me sympathetically and nodded several times, and I felt that he tried to understand me.

'I am really serious about it, and I would like to point out clearly once more that not a diet is concerned , but a radical change of my whole food to fruit and vegetables, and that I leave out all poisons known to me, like alcohol, coffee, tea, meat, bread and noodles. Moreover, I have not smoked anymore for 20 years already and do dumbbell training every day.'

My heart was pounding up to my collar. I had talked me into great excitement.

'What you do is right and admirable. But I know no patient who has kept this up. This is probably why there are no surveys about that. But if you could really reduce your creatinine values by this method, I would write a scientific report for our specialist journal.'

**Chapter 44**

The next morning began, as you could say, as usual. If you simply do not follow old habits anymore, new habits come inevitably. You should always also check these whether they withstand new findings or must also be further developed.

For breakfast – 'Frühstück', a strange German word which seemed more and more strange to me – I squeezed my oranges again, poured two grams of pure vitamin C in and drank it up slowly. I properly felt how the energy flowed out into my head.

It was another feeling than with coffee. I felt brighter in my brain and was immediately inspired to do something again.

Before showering I finished my dumbbell exercises.

This morning I made an incredible twelve repetitions. With a swollen breast, I went out of my room to the kitchen, where my wife was sitting with her cup of coffee and looked thoughtfully at the terrace.

'Twelve, I have made twelve repetitions,' I boasted. She looked up and said almost casually:

'Then you can help me clean the windows.'

That is how she was and is, but she did not mean this in any nasty way, but probably did not want excessive strength to remain unused. Window cleaning, hoovering, taking away the waste and gardening, those were my duties, and I used to like to stand in the kitchen and to prepare delicacies as well.

This happened frequently at weekends. The door to the terrace wide open, the sun was shining into the kitchen, the CD player filled the room with Spanish songs that made the sun look even brighter , and you believed to hear the sound of the sea and to taste the salt.

The ice cold white wine rounded the atmosphere to a paradisiacal state, which would even have brought Alfred Biolek into raptures. Escalope in cream sauce with paprika, enriched with creme fraiche, or beef olives not with bacon, but with fine smoked ham, smeared with Lyon mustard and creamy tomato sauce, thinly sliced cucumbers, etc. – pleasure was not a foreign word to me.

Today, in the morning when I got hungry for something edible, I grabbed a banana or an apple, and I wondered that this lasted until lunch. Later I would learn that in two apples more fibers are included than in a whole grain slice.

On this day, after talking to Dr Grevenbeck, there was cream herring from the market, of course from the Dutch stand, with jacket potatoes without salt and cucumber salad with olive oil and lemon.

In the last few days, I had thought about cancelling my shop and set up the child's room of our son, who had moved away, as an office.

Due to the fact that I now had no more trips to the office and back – meanwhile I always drove home at noon to go to bed for half an hour –, I had more time. Of course, Beate now wanted to fit me into the household more intensely, but a new habit developed that was not only emotionally good for us, but also brought me a lot of health benefits:

Walk.

And so we made our way in any weather, between office work and customer visits. If time permitted, we drove out by car and visited neighbouring cities or intentionally sought destinations.

The next day I had a customer visit near Winterswijk at the Dutch border. I decided to take Beate along and then stroll with her in this friendly small Dutch town.

I wanted to forget about the final laboratory report, or in any case I pretended to, but it was not to work. Persistent doubts came up to me whether I suffer from self-overestimation, which belonged to human nature since the evolution, and will inevitably die of kidney failure. Maybe the road I took is a dead end and I get fatally onto the wrong track?

The catastrophic lab report, the years of development of renal insufficiency, which then became chronic, the many other upsettingly threatening blood values, my increasing fatigue – my fear I could not explain away. I was well on the way to suppress my illness and distract myself against my better judgment.

**Chapter 45**

15th of October, 2010. A date which I will never again forget in my life.

Beate had taken part in the customer conversation, like when we had still ventured all appointments together, just like we had also finished all professional seminars together and had supported each other professionally.

We were a well-functioning team. In every customer conversation it is, regardless of the sales object, always about psychology and knowledge of human nature. Not only do you have to be authentic, but take the customer with their wishes and images seriously and honestly try to understand them.

If you are lucky, the customer forgives you for a mistake and you are corrected in a friendly way, but the 'shot can also immensely backfire'. A customer conversation carried on professionally is always very strenuous, and sometimes it is helpful to have somebody at your side with whom you can afterwards discuss the course of the conversation to avoid one or other mistake next time.

After such a conversation, which lasts, as a rule, one and a half hours, Beate and I often sat together and tried to analyse everything and everybody. However, today after the conversation with an older nice lady, we went over the border to Holland in the darkness and were quiet.

Holland. This other way of life exudes an undefinable peculiar holiday feeling. There were the houses without curtains, the people who went along the streets slower than where we live – everything looked much more relaxed than in Germany.

We parked in a byroad of a residential quarter and saved the parking fee. We liked to run through such streets and soaked up the other, lighter attitude to life in ourselves.

After a few minutes we reached the pedestrian zone and looked into the shop-windows that seemed almost ready for Christmas already. In Holland closing time is earlier than where we live, and the glass cabinets were decorated like in dollhouses, sometimes a little overloaded, but nevertheless tasteful, and also sometimes on the border of kitsch. We also relaxed noticeably and went more slowly. We unconsciously adapted to the deceleration of the Dutch strollers.

I felt exactly the opposite in myself – a tension like shortly before bursting, an internal cramping which could be felt even more clearly in this apparently lighter world of feeling. I stopped in front of a typical Dutch snack.

'I was born in Holland and raised in Germany, but the chips here, we don't have them, not like this. How I would like to eat such a thing once more! It cuts me to the quick when I inhale this smell, my mouth is watering. Come, let's go on and another way back. I cannot stand this here anymore.'

Beate nodded, and we turned back. In front of the small church, which reminded me of my old model railway church, the restaurants and cafés

139

were opened, the first radiant heaters were already put up, and young and old people excitedly were having a good time at the many small tables. The smells moved my stomach into a mine field. This was not endurable. I turned to my wife, and we disappeared in an empty byroad without shops.

'Your mobile phone is ringing!' Beate shouted. I had not assigned the ringing tone to my mobile phone. It had almost never rung during the last few days. I rummaged about awkwardly in the jacket pocket, and really, there really rang my mobile phone.

'Hello,' I breathed into the tiny black mike, 'hello?'

'This is Grevenbeck speaking.' My breath caught, my heart pounded like a hammer against my lower jaw, my hands trembled.

'Yes?'

It was no more that came from my throat. Then I heard the other voice again, the voice of Dr Grevenbeck:

'I know that it is quite late and it is Friday evening. But I wanted to inform you of it absolutely immediately. I was so glad for you.'

Now I understood nothing at all anymore.

'Sorry?'

- nothing more was possible.

'Your creatinine level. I have just received your lab value by fax. Your creatinine level is again down to two point eight!'

'Thanks, thanks, thanks,' I pressed the red spot and started to cry - in the middle on the street.

## Chapter 46

I had gone on some steps alone with the mobile phone in my ear . Now I turned round, saw Beate, swept up both arms and shouted: 'Yeeeees!'

It made no difference to me whether somebody saw me – or shook their head, thought I was mad. But nobody was there – except Beate. She stared at me, surprised:

'What happened, tell me already!'

'That was Dr Grevenbeck,' I shouted. I could not calm down, my body trembled, and I opened the zipper of my jacket with a jerk. I needed air.

'My creatinine level is down, to two point eight, the lab report is already there. I don't know, I can't tell you at all … I think today I have been born all over again. Now I have two birthdays.'

I turned away from her to hide my tears. In my whole life I had never been so glad. I breathed deeply several times. She embraced me and pressed me quite firmly to herself. I slowly calmed down, but I remained agitated and excited. I could not understand it. Somehow it did not want to get into my head. I tried desperately to remember the date when I was with Dr von Rothenburg, when he reported to me about the high kidney value and then sent me to the dialysis clinic.

'Do you still know when I was at the family doctor's and he had informed me of the creatinine value?' I asked in a shaking voice. I wanted to calm down again with all my might, become normal, appear quiet.

'Yes, I believe this was the 7th of September,' she answered without stopping to chew on the chewing gum.

'Why do you ask?'

'Exactly one week later I started eating only fruit, and the following Sunday, we flew to Majorca.' I started to count in my head.

'On the 15th of September I started eating fruit. So more or less exactly four weeks were sufficient. This is astonishing. Even I did not count on that. From four point one, one back to two point eight. I still can't believe it.'

I shook my head and, doing that, looked to the ground.

'Cheer up, a new life is starting now', and her voice became high, as usual when she was glad. She took my left hand, and we went back to the city centre.

I stopped jerkily in front of the snack.

'You know what, now I'll get chips, with mayonnaise. That's what I deserve. I will now allow this to myself.'

I let go of her hand and walked into the salesroom as if to an award ceremony.

## Chapter 47

The journey back nearly took 2.5 hours. I have never gone so slowly. I still trembled internally. It had been dark for a long time already.

'I cannot grasp it yet,' I whispered.

Beate understood, nevertheless, and said:

'This just goes to show what difference food makes if you avoid all poisons.'

'Unfortunately, I must confess something to you.'

She turns her head in my direction.

'What's the matter?'

'I slowly get aches in my stomach.'

'You shouldn't have eaten the chips.'

'But I had been so looking forward to it. You cannot imagine at all how ravenously hungry I was for such a thing. I basically wanted to feel like I used to. Preferably I would still have drunk a beer in addition. But I could only just keep this back.'

'Then you would feel quite rotten now, I can assure you.'

'I believe, I must stop for a bit and walk a few metres.'

I drove into a lay-by and got out. Beate remained seated in the car. In my stomach everything seemed to turn, like in a washing machine. Acid climbed up somehow, and I felt a disagreeable taste in my mouth. I did not feel like vomiting at all. I went slowly, but without stopping, along the dark country road. There were no lanterns, and the sky released its glittering stars. The fresh autumn air was good for me. After a while I turned round and found out that the car had shrunk to Matchbox size. I slowly went back. Beate had already been worried. She felt that I came to terms better alone at such moments.

'Better?'

'Yes, I'm OK again. It was worth the experience.'

'You are all white in your face and have bluish red bags under your eyes. This must have battered you quite a lot.'

'As soon as we are home, I must drink water. I already feel now that this will be good for me.'

'Just stop at the next filling station,' she suggested.

'It's OK again,' I answered. I opened the side window and breathed deeply.

'No stranger will believe me this, that you can be so devastated by chips. For me this was like pure poison. If I only remember, I'm feeling sick.'

'I don't like eating such fat stuff anyway, but you have always liked to eat chips, particularly the Dutch ones. This is quite astonishing how the body adapts itself if it is used only to the best things.'

I could only agree to this by nodding.

I could not imagine on this evening that my experiences were not finished with the present day yet.

## Chapter 48

Professional stress completely controlled me fast again, and I desperately thought about how I could avoid these continuous excessive demands. I had to continue attending to my present customers, of course, but I looked for future alternatives. From my experience of long years I was aware that problems take long to be solved. Then, however, the solution comes mostly all of a sudden. It is vital that you always remain on the ball and do not surrender, always look round yourself where possibilities open.

Human beings are by nature impatient and always want everything preferably immediately. I am convinced that you can practice patience. First you should exactly tell yourself or even write down at which target you aim. You will then also keep this in your head more easily. Doing that, you may not neglect your current occupation. However, in addition I wanted to nourish myself optimally, and a feeling spread slowly that I would like to call carelessness.

Some days after my Holland trip I was on the way to a customer again. I heard some tiresome small talk on the radio, and my thoughts went to the preparation of a lunch.

I used to like cooking. Basically I would even do it still today, but I have changed my habits radically, after all. Nevertheless, I catch myself over and over again as I think of the preparation of food. I made clear to myself in my thoughts over and over again what it actually is what you eat. One of these bewildering terms was the word starch. Who does not want to be strong? But the word leads us into a wrong direction.

It is not long ago what I had read in Wikipedia on the subject starch:

While warming up starch, in particular in baking, frying and roasting in the presence of the amino acid asparagine, the carcinogene acrylamide may develop.

And then there was still the starch slime which deposits in the body and in the long term causes discomfort like knee pain, rheumatism and stiffness etc. due to eating bread.

I had become aware of that long ago. However, this knowledge collided with my recollection that I felt so good, that food, particularly my self-prepared one, was very tasty, it already smelt enticingly in preparation.

I imperceptibly distracted myself from the traffic and only woke again properly when I stood in front of the house of the customer. I actually had wanted to refuel as well. I had completely forgotten about this.

When I drive off again afterwards, I'll absolutely have to go directly to a filling station.

I looked at the tank indicator through the steering wheel. It was down to the ground, and the controlling lamp glowed. I looked at the kilometre reading and read 195273.

Next to it was the indicator how many kilometres I could still go: seven. This could just barely work, I thought. The next filling station is very near, after all. OK.

Then the usual grip into the breast pocket for my reading glasses, and off to the customer. However, I remained seated as if petrified. Something was different. What had happened? I was irritated.

Then the scales literally fell from the eyes. I read the kilometre readings – without reading glasses. Unbelievable! I shook my head, almost quivering, and would not believe it. Maybe I even only fantasized and have not yet woken at all. I was sitting here, after all, here in the car. That was reality.

I looked at the kilometre reading again. Really 195273. I reached for the mobile phone. Beate's number was stored.

'It's me.'

'Has anything happened? You have only just driven off!'

'No. Yes. Everything is all right. I just wanted to inform you immediately that I can look again', I shouted into the receiver.

'Humph. What do you mean, look?'

She must have thought I was off my trolley. I smiled about my 'polished communication'.

'Yes. I look at the kilometre reading and can read the figures – without reading glasses. My visual strength has changed, so properly, so obviously, as the word says, improved. I can see better. I cannot grasp it.'

'Although you have not eaten all that many carrots.'

'You don't have to make fun at all. I just wanted to tell you right away.'

'This is not so unusual at all. I can remember that with optimum food one can also see clearer. But I don't know anymore where I read this.'

'So take care, see you soon.'

I hung up and minced light-footedly to the front door of the customer, read his name without glasses and rang.

**Chapter 49**

As a schoolboy I had already done odd jobs. In our town there had been in my youth an intra-urban zoo with a so-called zoo restaurant. You could look from the dining room directly at the red deer enclosure, even when venison ragout was on the menu.

I will never forget some looks of guests who pounced on their meat with relish and how their throat contracted when they noticed the living animals of the same name of the menu. Deer, particularly the young, have wonderful amber-coloured, sloping eyes which look so affectionately at you that you become deeply moved. You cannot avoid such looks.

In the afternoon, in any case, there was always cake of the finest quality. We, the waiters, were allowed to swallow up separate oddments, and we were always hungry. And I learnt to drink coffee. Later during my studies and in my job as well I did not like to renounce my piece of cake in the afternoon, preferably Black Forest Cherry or Cream Cheese, and coffee. Because I had always been sporty and in our town the bicycle had a special value, I have also never gained weight. And now, now I had already drunk no coffee and had eaten no cake for three months.

It was the 2nd of November, 2010, when I became weak and was to remain weak. The lab report had come. There it was written in black and white: creatinine two point eight. I got the first lab report and, with my low knowledge, compared the other figures.

Also all the other blood values had moved into the healthier direction. I was more than content. I was happy, and I wanted to treat myself to something, but no chips.

Cake became the object of desire, and coffee. Espresso was said to be healthier than normally brewed up coffee. November had already completely struck, the sky was grey, but it did not rain.

This afternoon no more customer appointment was pending, and so I used the opportunity to invite Beate to the market café. Cream Cheese and an espresso. My mouth watered. I used to drink coffee only black and without sugar, even more so at the time when I was still smoking, or as they say nowadays, when smoking was still healthy.

'Oh Beate, I don't smoke, haven't done so for more than seventeen years already, I drink no wine, no beer, eat no meat and almost no flour-based dishes. I think that I should treat myself to coffee and cake once. What do you think?'

'Can coffee be a sin?' she hummed with the well-known melody.

'You were so consistent up to now. I think you will not die of it. Nevertheless, it always remains your decision. We have talked very often already about the fact that in life you must always decide, every day anew. And if new knowledge is added, it should also be incorporated. It always gets dramatic when decisions are made which you don't recognise as such at all, but act without knowing. You expose yourself to an external influence, a foreign control if you do not carefully examine your decisions, particularly the important ones in life, and always revaluate them. You should always be aware of the criteria according to which you choose your decisions. The values are vital. The values of life. I must always ask myself: Is this good for me, for others, is this good or bad?'

'Coffee is not good for me. Coffee is a poison and attacks the kidneys, which then go crazy and put the whole body on alert. This is also why you suddenly become wide awake,' I complemented competently.

I sprinkled plenty of sugar into the espresso and drank it slowly, but in one go.

It was a thrillingly great feeling.

**Chapter 50**

For weeks I have been doing my dumbbell exercises every morning and every evening . Consistently. Meanwhile they already take up to 10 minutes. November became dank, and I felt no desire at all to go for a walk in my spare time, although the fresh air was always very good for me. I still remember exactly how I stood in front of my dumbbells one morning and said loudly to myself:

'Today you will crack one hundred.'

I took the 5-kilo dumbbells and began with the repetitions. From ninety I had to torment myself. With 98 my biceps seemed to burst. Funnily enough, I made 100 quite easily. I beamed and hurried, in my underpants, to the kitchen, where Beate was sitting with her usual mug of coffee, looked at the terrace and thought.

'I made 100,' I shouted excitedly.

'You know what, I need heavier dumbbells. They are just too lightweight. One should not do so many repetitions at all, but less, but with more weight instead.'

'I wouldn't be surprised either if sometime you're going to enroll to the Olympic Games,' she smiled.

'But I should also do something once again. I would feel like going swimming once again. To the sole swimming-pool, that would be something, what do you think?'

'I would also like this, but you're giving me another idea there. I used to like playing indoor football and volleyball. Whether I can still play volleyball at almost 60, however, with the new rules, I am very uncertain. However, football, this would maybe work.'


I quickly drank my orange juice with two grams of vitamin C and ran to the shower. When later I was sitting at my computer, I looked for sports clubs in town which also offered indoor football. It was quite a strange feeling when I entered my date of birth and the word senior citizen's sport appeared. I accepted this awful truth and really found a team of players over thirty who always met on Tuesdays, at eight o'clock in the evening, in a small suburban hall. I knew the area and decided not to call, but to go there simply.

I could still go swimming, but today is Tuesday. I rummaged about in the wardrobe. I had no sports bag at all. A shopping bag of Beate's was to help out, and the old sneakers, I smirked, would excite in the sports museum. But I took them nevertheless. Sports trousers were also found, but no jersey. An old T-shirt should also be enough. I needed only 10 minutes to the hall by car.

The hall door was locked, and I rang. A slender, well-trained older man in a well-groomed tracksuit opened, looked at me from top to bottom, scrutinising, and asked:
'Can I help?'

I explained to him that I had found out on the internet that maybe one can play football here et cetera, in any case, I was standing in the hall in no time at all and was put into the team of my door opener.

This was suitable, because now two teams were confronted four against four. The interior parts of boxes formed the small goals, the rules were as formerly, and off we went. After a few minutes already I found myself on the bench. Not that I would have been disqualified, no, I could not do it anymore. I was completely out of breath. After the first breather I ran again for some minutes. Thus it went the whole hour. Finally, I was finished. I received consolation from all partners and was invited to come again.

'And on Thursdays we play volleyball.' The only body movement which I still managed painlessly was a nod.

## Chapter 51

Football on Tuesdays, volleyball on Thursdays, this was already an immense increase compared to former times. At football I was the youngest at the age of 58 years, at volleyball sports friends from the football squad of Tuesday were also present, but there were also some younger players. I used to stay in clubs a lot, and the atmosphere also was as it used to be. They quite made a point of being present regularly. That was also good, because this light social pressure transformed the appointments into a certain routine.

We simply went to football on Tuesdays because it was Tuesday, and we went to volleyball on Thursdays because it was Thursday. Otherwise the joy in playing together predominated. From time to time they mixed the same groups, and with some repetitions of these oppositions, sport competitions developed.

There were, in between or in the fitting room, opportunities over and over again to speak to each other, to exchange experiences and to get to know each other more closely. Some footballers were already far over 70 and one even over eighty years old. The group had been managed for over thirty years by a former sports teacher who had co-founded the group at the time.

I admired these older teammates. Although they were around twenty years older, they were fitter than I was. For weeks I had to fight with muscle ache, but I hung on. I felt how I got closer and closer to the performance of the older ones and was also supported by everyone and was recognised in my endeavours.

Years ago I had once begun an attempt to take physical exercise and had gone to a fitness centre, a so-called muscle factory. In the beginning it was new and had even been a little fun. But it became more and more dull, and I felt more and more lonely on the devices. Sometime I did not go any longer. However, I still paid my monthly contributions for it for more than a year.

Of course I had not forgotten that Beate wanted to go swimming with me. When she noticed how good the organized sport was for me, she also wanted to search a group for herself, maybe something with dancing. In any case, one day, we went to the sole bath in the Ruhr area after all. It was a big bath with a holiday atmosphere, several basins with different temperature in the inside area, but also a very big basin with a view of the engraving plant, filled with sea water from the depths of the sole.

It was more than 30 degrees warm and steamed. In the dusk, an almost uncanny atmosphere was generated. Only the heads and the bright steam, which evaporated into the dark sky, could be seen. Inside there was also a café, a sauna and relaxation rooms.

We had put together two sun loungers for us and curled up in the warm room with artificial palms.

I laid my arms over my head and crossed them in my nape. My chest lifted, and my shoulder joints came to their limit of stretching. I stopped short and turned to my nicer half on the left:

'Have a look how far I can stretch again. And it doesn't hurt at all. This is phenomenal.'

She bent over to me and said:

'Yes, you have really become more agile, but just show your forearms.'

I sat upright and stretched my arms towards her. I had so burnt my forearms sometime on a boat trip in the Mediterranean Sea that for many years already I wore long-sleeved shirts also in summer. They would start to burn immediately if the sun stroked them just a little. What Beate had noticed also surprised me: On one hand, the skin was not all that dark anymore, the borders to the healthy skin not so strong in contrast anymore, rather blurred, and on the darker skin many small white spots had formed.

'Your skin seems to regenerate. You are slowly starting to creep me out, with your healthy food.'

## Chapter 52

The days became shorter, and so I sat in front of the PC more often and looked further for information worth knowing. The internet is inexhaustible and can properly addict.

'You're sitting in front of the box again. On which search are you now then?' Beate asked, standing in the door entrance.

'I have already made such a lot of progress, but I simply can't get away from one thing. Again and again it is stressed in the most different versions that vegetarians must face deficiency symptoms if they eat no meat or meat products at all. Now I'm looking for scientific investigations which give me information about the ingredients. But I can't find such a list anywhere which vitamins, amino acids and so on are in fruit or meat and bread,' I answered and dully went on googling.

'Knowing you as I do, you will study biochemistry rather than surrender. On television there is a crime thriller from Münster, but as I notice, you'd rather continue.'

She was not miffed, but she would rather have had me with herself.

Then under 'ein-langes-leben.de' I find the sentence: '… taurine and carnitine (both amino acids) … are other nutrients which are often absent in the vegan raw food.'

So, a lack in raw food after all?

I enter taurine in Wikipedia, and there is written:

'The adult human body can produce *taurine* of the amino acid cysteine itself.'

Then I enter carnitine and find:

'The human body can form L-carnitine from the amino acids methionine and lysine itself, but takes it up primarily through meat.'

And that is the limit by all means, I think when I read that taurine and carnitine are no amino acids at all as had been maintained in the first text. I cannot shake the suspicion that one tries with every trick in the book, consciously or uninformedly, to insinuate deficiency symptoms as a result of vegetarian as well as vegan food.

I looked further under amino acids in Wikipedia:

'Amino acids which an animal organism needs, but cannot produce itself, are called essential amino acids and must be taken up with the food…. For human beings valine, methionine, leucine, isoleucine, phenylalanine, tryptophane, threonine and lysine are essential amino acids. … The remaining amino acids are either directly synthesised or are gained from other amino acids by modification.' Etc.

The other amino acids are not essential and can be produced by the body itself: These are, according to Wikipedia, among others:

'Arginine, asparagine, cysteine, glutamine, glycine, proline, tyrosine, alanine, glutamate, uric acid, histidine and serine.'

Now I am neither a doctor, nor a biochemist, but I am now interested in knowing which of these amino acids are in fruit and which are absent. These cannot be vitamins, of course. It is clear that meat has not got all vitamins, but these are found in particular in fruit and vegetables.

Through impossible ways I have bumped on www.kochrezepte.de, and there they were all listed, all 20 amino acids, and all are in apples, you do not believe it, but also all vitamins, all trace elements, all carbohydrates and all fibres are listed. Unfortunately, this page was taken down again, for whatever reason. But there are still other tips as well, as for example: www.gesundheit.de/ernaehrung/lebensmittel/obst/apfel.

But all ingredients of all kinds of meat were also listed, and even more still. All that was not even written in Wikipedia. After my experience so far and my dilettantish smattering of knowledge, the suspicion suggests itself to me that for decades, vegetarians, let alone vegans, have been threatened with deficiency symptoms in their food, while it is rather the other way round, that meat eaters much more likely run the risk of not supplying themselves sufficiently with all nutrients.

Now I also remember that sometime an experiment had been cancelled in America after some two weeks, where students had lived only on meat. The cancellation had become necessary because they would otherwise have died.

I must absolutely speak to Beate of my suspicion of decades of twist of reality in favour of meat consumption. I ran into the sitting room and found her asleep on the couch, no wonder, it was already half past two.

**Chapter 53**

Christmas. Christmas Eve. Last year Beate's children, 23 and 24 years old meanwhile, were with their friends on Christmas Eve, or with their parents together with them, and had visited us on the first Christmas Day. This year it was to be the other way round. Today both children wanted to come to us.

What do you make for dinner then? Apples, oranges and nuts are healthy and Christmas omnipresent. We decided on potato salad without meat, different kinds of fish, garnished in small morsels, and colourful salads, enriched with pistachios and grapes.

We had just covered the round table when the doorbell already rang.

I had wished for new dumbbells, otherwise my wife and I had been giving each other nothing for a long time anymore already, but saved everything for the children. Age plays no role there. You are always happy when the children are happy - even if they have grown for a long time, they remain children -, and thus Beate manages every year anew to hide many small surprises in lots of wrapping paper to let the joy of giving away continue for as long as possible.

'Go on laying the table, I'll open already,' she shouted, and I got the glasses from the cupboard, wineglasses for fresh spring water.

Philipp, taller than I by a head, stamped directly to me with his thick, fatty leather boots and hugged me as usual. We like each other since I got the chance of knowing him at the age of seven years. As if by request, the doorbell rang again.

'That's what I call timing,' I whispered to Philipp.

'Otherwise, Svenja likes to come one hour later sometimes, but maybe she also wants to leave again earlier,' I reckoned a little sarcastically, but not seriously.

'She also has a new friend after all, you must understand this,' Philipp exculpated his sister whom he always protected as a matter of course.

'Hello, Svenja!' I shouted in the direction of the hallway: 'Merry Christmas, come in, it's getting cold.'

I was still standing in the sitting room, Beate came through the door, switched off the big light and pulled Svenja into the room with her right hand. I did not trust my eyes. On her arms she carried a black-brown shaggy dog puppy like a baby. The small snub nose aimed at me and the big eyes ate me up.

'You have bought yourself a dog? You're still studying after all. Oh, doesn't matter. You will have thought about this. You will make it. But it is a lot of work. You know, we used to have a dachshund. You must look after a dog quite intensely. What's his name then?'

I noticed how Beate rolled her eyes.

'Well,' I said. 'I didn't mean it that way, sorry, and what's his name?'
Svenja smiled over all four cheeks, her big eyes which resembled her mother very much, shone in the dim light.

'Mila, a hybrid bitch, half a dachshund, half a Jack Russel, here, take her once.' She stretched the ball of wool against me. I just could not help holding my hands under it and taking up the little animal.
'Isn't she sweet?' she asked me directly.
'Well, that's how puppies are,' I replied, a little embarrassed.
'She is for you, for Christmas, for your kidneys. You have to go to the fresh air and go for a walk a lot after all.'

My family had probably never experienced me so taken aback, confused and nonplussed. I only shook my head, slowly sat down on my favorite arm-chair and no longer understood what was going on:
'I never wanted a dog again, though,' I whispered.
'But now you have one,' all three shouted as in one voice. Then Philipp brought a cuddly dog basket,

Svenja dragged small coloured bowls and bags with dog food into the room.

'Did you know about this?' I asked, looking to Beate. She shook her head:

'No, this is as surprising for me as for you.

But one thing I tell you, we won't give her away anymore. My God, is she cuddly!'

She took the little animal from me and pressed it quite firmly to her maternal breast.

'This is going to be fun,' I quietly spoke into the room.

'What should I say to that?'

'Preferably nothing at all,' reckoned Philipp and sat down near Beate on the couch.

'Svenja,' she suddenly said, in a strangely serious tone. She still had the animal in both hands and just wanted to give it over to Philipp, and now lifted it even higher:

'This is no female, this is a male dog. Look here.'

Svenja got closer:

'And I thought this was the belly button.'

„Then we'll simply call him Milan instead of Mila,' Philipp immediately came to the rescue.

'Milan is peeing,' shouted Beate suddenly, Philipp jumped up and bumped against the table so that the glasses wavered.

'Merry Christmas,' I heckled, 'this is a great start.'

## Chapter 54

One year has passed meanwhile. It is 2012. The lab reports prove that many blood values slowly improved further, and the most important value of all, the creatinine value, had remained steady. The chronic renal insufficiency had not progressed further, but remained stable at the diminished value of around 3.

As my family doctor supposed, my iron depot was very probably filled up to the brim, but the kidney was still not capable of exploiting the iron accordingly. This was also the real reason why, after a few hours of strain, whether physically or mentally, I became a little tired.

However, I felt fit as never before in my life. I neglected the dumbbell training quite a lot of times, though, but instead I went for a walk with the dog four times a day and regularly went to play football on Tuesdays and volleyball on Thursdays.

I did not need a breather every few minutes anymore, but strictly played through the one and a half hours each time.

I had maintained my food change, with the small weakness that I drank a cup of coffee in the morning and allowed myself a piece of cake on quite a lot of afternoons.

In some food stores freshly pressed orange juice in bottles had been available for some time. This meant I was not forced to have to squeeze oranges anymore.

Furthermore I enriched the daily glass of orange juice with one gram of vitamin C from the inexpensive 100-gram tin for just under three euros.

Alcohol, meat and wheat bread continued to be an absolute taboo. From time to time I could be enticed to a small pizza or vegetarian lasagna. If I visited a restaurant with friends, I first ordered a fruit plate and then a mixed salad with lemon dressing.

Cellagon as a food supplement had been recommended to me by a friend, a nutritional adviser. I had the feeling that this pure natural product from a comprehensive vitamin arrangement was good for me in addition.

In any case, my immune system must have become enormously strong. It had to be causally the immune system, otherwise the following healings were not to be explained:

It was in spring, 2013. I sat at the breakfast table and told my wife that I felt toothache when toothbrushing. I opened my mouth and raised the upper lip with the fingers. She got a proper fright and took me into the bathroom.

What I saw there in the mirror did not surprise me less: The whole gums of the lower jaw were bluish red and inflamed all around.

I was to go to the doctor immediately. I also wanted to keep the appointment with the dentist the next day. Only I had no more pains in the morning. The redness and the inflammation had completely disappeared. I cancelled the doctor's appointment and had no more discomfort since then.

By the winter I repaired the small garden house. The roof had become leaking. I spent the whole day kneeling on the roof and laid new roof tiles and bitumen panels. On the following Sunday I could neither run nor sit nor lie with pain in the knees. At night I shouted with pain so much that my wife wanted to call the emergency doctor.

On Monday the pain and knee inflammations were almost gone, and on Tuesday I played volleyball again. My self-healing forces had seemingly rebuilt themselves.

Since I administer myself the daily overdose of vitamin C, I did not have a trace of a cold or influenza. My walks with Milan extended to kilometres of long wanderings. The small dog has understandably got used to the many walks, Beate and I would not be so happy without them any more.

### In the end

'All thoughts are a function of our misery. If we understand certain things, the merit is exclusively due to certain defects of our health.'

The existential philosopher E. M. Cioran wrote this sentence in his book *'The New Gods'*.

Only when you become ill, have suffered an accident, you come to appreciate the healthy state. It is a phenomenon that you do not feel health. If you are healthy and you sit, for example, in a comfortable armchair, you should sometimes close your eyes and try to feel yourself.

The body is full of nerves, bones, joints, muscles and organs, and you feel nothing. The body does not seem to be there at all, as if it was completely transparent.

Only pain changes our behaviour and our attitude towards the body with a lasting effect, because we not only have a body, but we are a body.

The disastrous thing in a kidney disease is now that you have no pain in the beginning. Even if you become fatter and fatter or you smoke or drink your little glass of wine every day, you notice nothing, even less so if you are young.

The problem is the slow imperceptible poisoning. Constant dripping wears the stone. For twenty, thirty or forty years we regularly consume food with additives with the known or rather unknown E numbers, every day we eat bread with the glue material, every day we eat meat and sausage with growth hormones and antibiotics and many other poisons, more or less every day we drink the smallest parts of nerve poison in the form of alcohol, every day we consume convenience food with a massive, well disguised portion of sugar and/or salt in an amount which goes way beyond the healthy level.

I am not surprised anymore that so many people, millions and millions in the western world, die of cancer, kidney failure and cardiac infarction. There has never been in the history of humanity such a long phase of so-called prosperity like the last 50, 60 years. The selection in food is so gigantic that a single person is properly demanded too much. In a medium-sized shop around 60,000 different articles of food are offered.

I have already got used to passing in all deliberateness the dozens of shelves without always only shaking my head. In an earlier chapter I had already pointed out that shops with displays of fresh fruit, luminous oranges and lemons attract the people, such as in Germany in the supermarkets there is always first the fruit and vegetable department built up.

This is a clue for the fact that people feel by nature attracted by sweet fruit and must have lived, at the beginning of the history of mankind, essentially on fruits. Their digestive organs are designed for fruit consumption.

But why do people poison themselves visibly?

Food manufacturers are not meanwhile called food industry for no reason. It is gigantic, and a turnover of thousands of millions is had worldwide. I do not begrudge all involved parties their salary and profit, but these already go at the expense of health.

168

Bad eating habits are developed and stabilised with the help of thousands of millions in advertising.

Quite apart from the fact that here legislation is also challenged, people are subject to the tasty seduction and erroneously think that variety and amount make prosperity.

Adults will not change their bad, unhealthy habits so fast, but they have the moral obligation to lead their children to a more deliberate nutrition. In this point most parents and the school fail. Moreover, you can extensively retrieve information on the Internet, make yourself smart. But without consciousness people rather chat about nonsense for hours or play computer games until they drop.

Only with consciousness, moral action arises, and with responsible action, consciousness arises. Where should you begin there?

In the end, everyone is responsible for themselves. Nearly two years had to pass until I could write down my 'story'. I was thereby forced to confront myself again with my fears at that time. However, I believe it was worthwhile. Over and over again I had been asked by friends and acquaintances to write a small book about it, with the aim to encourage others and to show that you can change something.

In writing, it struck me that I have not once taken up the concept which I have heard much too often from others in this connection:

'It is difficult to overcome your weaker self.'

I did not have this internal weakness, and I am convinced that it is just another excuse to deal intensely with one's own erratic behaviour. This requires laborious thinking and difficult retraining and with it always an overcoming of fear.

This fear runs deep, and you would not like to lose your face. Also you do not want to position yourself outside of society. But there are more and more people who are on the way to desire to live in a healthier way. This gave me courage and confidence to be respected on a continuing basis, also or even especially as a fruit eater, non-smoker, teetotaller and someone who avoids meat.

I for one have escaped from the last stage, the life-menacing stage IV of the chronic renal insufficiency, and have brought the chronic renal insufficiency to a stop. I quote at this point from www.curado.de/Niereninsuffizienz-Therapie-10590:

'However, in the final stage of a chronic renal insufficiency, an artificial cleaning of the blood by dialysis is mostly unavoidable.'

I have consistently released my kidneys from the work to filter out toxins, so that they can recover. This alone the professional world has disavowed as virtually impossible. On account of my nutrition, which is extremely free of poison, the chronically diseased kidneys are perceptibly relieved. I am certainly not cured, but not on dialysis either. Now I live free of pain and hope to stay untroubled by dialysis for as long as possible this way.

My blood values are almost normal again after two years. I am physically fit and exceptionally well-trained. I experience the overwhelming feeling to be painless and virtually healthy on a daily basis. I feel light, and my head is bright and clear.

As Goethe said, thus or alike:

'What use has a lot of money to the people,
no sick person enjoys the world.'

Lab notes:

Here are the demonstrable creatinine values of the extensive lab examinations:

4th Oct. 2010 mg/dl creatinine 4.11

2nd Nov. 2010 mg/dl creatinine 2.8

2nd Nov. 2011 mg/dl creatinine 3.0

## Literary references and Internet sites:

www.curado.de

www.symptome.ch

www.dialyse-online.de

www.med4you.at

www.kochrezepte.de

www.youtube.de: Wie ich der Dialyse entkam...

Dieter Reinecker

Helmut Wandmaker: Rohkost statt Feuertopf,
Goldmann Verlag, ISBN 978-3-442-13912-5

E.M. Cioran: Die verfehlte Schöpfung,
Suhrkamp Verlag,

ISBN 978-3-518-37050-6

Note:

For reasons of data protection, the names of the doctors were replaced by fictitious names.